All About

Prostate Cancer

FRED STEPHENS

AM MD MS FRCS(Ed) FACS FRACS
Professor Emeritus and former Head,
Department of Surgery,
University of Sydney;
Consultant Emeritus in Surgical Oncology,
Sydney Hospital and Royal Prince Alfred
Hospital, Sydney, Australia

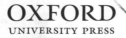

OXFORD
UNIVERSITY PRESS

OXFORD
UNIVERSITY PRESS

253 Normanby Road, South Melbourne, Victoria, Australia

Oxford University Press is a department of the University of Oxford.
It furthers the University's objective of excellence in research, scholarship,
and education by publishing worldwide in

Oxford New York

Athens Auckland Bangkok Bogotá
Buenos Aires Calcutta Cape Town Chennai
Dar es Salaam Delhi Florence Hong Kong
Istanbul Karachi Kuala Lumpur Madrid Melbourne
Mexico City Mumbai Nairobi Paris Port Moresby
São Paulo Shanghai Singapore Taipei Tokyo Toronto Warsaw
and associated companies in
Berlin Ibadan

OXFORD is a trade mark of Oxford University Press

National Library of Australia
Cataloguing-in-publication data:

Stephens, Frederick Oscar.
   All about prostate cancer.

   Bibliography.
   Includes index.
   ISBN 0 19 551404 1.

   1. Prostate—Cancer. I. Title.

616.65

Edited by Elaine Cochrane
Indexed by Russell Brooks
Cover designed by MAPG
Typeset by Solo Typesetting, South Australia
Printed through Bookpac Production Services, Singapore

All About

Prostate Cancer

Foreword

Just after I had been told by the urologist that I had prostate cancer, I proceeded to drive the full length of a one-way street in the wrong direction. I didn't even hear the car horns and the irate shouts!

I have since discovered that many men behave in a similar irrational manner when they are first told that they've got 'it'. This reaction is caused not just by shock at the diagnosis, but also by confusion at the bewildering array of medical solutions presented, all of them surrounded by question marks. To be suddenly confronted by coloured diagrams of the inner workings of the male anatomy, together with often incomprehensible words and medical techniques, and to know that they all refer directly to you, tends to leave the average bloke totally confused, very frightened, and most of all terribly lonely. The confusion is compounded because at the end of the consultation most men are asked to go away and decide for themselves which of the different treatment options presented they wish to undertake.

Now, at last, we have a book setting out the whole thing in layman's language yet written by an expert. Professor Stephens has spent a great deal of his life researching, understanding and explaining the mysteries of this disease, and he explains it with remarkable simplicity and frankness. His in-depth knowledge, together with his sympathetic understanding of where the patient is coming from, makes this volume an absolute must for men and their families. I believe the greater the partner's understanding, the more the partner can assist in the decision-making, and this support can take away an enormous part of the loneliness.

Prostate cancer is not a death sentence. It can be defeated, and understanding your enemy goes a long way towards achieving the victory. I therefore commend this book in the highest possible terms. It is a medical book for non-medicos. And aren't most of us just that?

Roger Climpson
Patron, Prostate Cancer Research Foundation of Australia

Dedication

This book is dedicated to my alma mater, the University of Sydney, and especially to past and present colleagues and friends in the Department of Surgery. The University and Faculty of Medicine paid me the great honour of appointing me to a personal Chair in Surgery and Surgical Oncology, and my friends and colleagues in the Department of Surgery paid me a considerable honour in electing me their chief.

I dedicate this book also to my wonderful family and extended family, and especially to the memory of my much-loved late brother Stan, who battled this cancer with courage and dignity.

Dedication

Contents

Illustrations

Tables

Tables

Acknowledgments

I am grateful to a number of friends, colleagues and members of my family for advice, particularly in what they thought should be in this book and on whether my descriptions and writings were clear to them. Dr John Rogers, Senior Urological Surgeon of the Royal Prince Alfred Hospital and President of the Urological Society of Australia, Dr Michael Boyer, Head of the Department of Medical Oncology at the Royal Prince Alfred Hospital, and Professor Alan Coates, Chairman of the Australian Cancer Society, were particularly helpful regarding the contents, as was Dr Graham Stevens, Head of Radiation Oncology at the Royal Prince Alfred Hospital. Mr Roger Climpson, Patron of the Prostate Cancer Research Foundation of Australia, paid me the compliment of writing a foreword for this book from a patient's point of view.

As always, my friend (and Australia's prominent radio and media doctor) Dr James Wright was full of helpful suggestions in arranging publication. My dear wife Sheilagh, who is a lecturer in literacy at the University of Technology, Sydney, is my constant adviser and critic of all my writings. Sheilagh's sister, Frances Kelly, who is a literary agent, and her brother Kieran Kelly also read the manuscript and gave encouraging and helpful advice.

Mr Bob Haynes, of the Royal Prince Alfred Hospital Medical Illustrations Department, turned my rough illustrations into well-drawn art, and Dr Andrew McLaughlin, of the Royal Prince Alfred Hospital Nuclear Medicine Department, kindly provided the bone scan illustrations.

Mr Peter Rose of Oxford University Press was most helpful in arranging publication of this book, and I am grateful to Ms Elaine Cochrane for her work in editing the manuscript.

$$\left(\begin{array}{c}1\end{array}\right)$$

What is the prostate?

The prostate or prostate gland is an essential component of the male sexual structure, not only of humans but also of all male mammals, from elephants and whales to mice and kangaroos.

In men the prostate is a small gland about the size of a walnut that is in the lower pelvis just below the bladder. It is composed of between 20 and 30 small glands surrounded by and joined by tissue containing muscle fibres. The back of the gland can be felt by a doctor carrying out what is called a PR (per rectum) or DRE (digital rectal examination) by inserting a finger in the anus. In

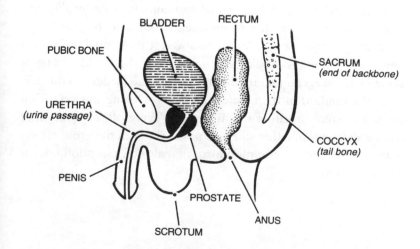

Figure 1.1 The position and anatomy of the prostate gland.

front of the prostate is the pubic bone (felt at the top of the penis) and behind it is the lower rectum and anus.

The prostate lies on a sling or hammock of muscles that stretch from one side of the pelvis to the other. It is surrounded by a rich network of blood vessels, and because it is in a small contained space behind the pubic bone, below the bladder and in front of the rectum and anus, operations in this area are difficult and require special surgical skills and techniques.

The prostate becomes larger as men grow older. By the age of 40, about 30 per cent of men will have some degree of enlargement of their prostates. By 60, about 50 per cent will have some prostate enlargement, and at the age of 80 nearly all men will have an enlarged prostate.

The urethra, the passage for urine to pass from the bladder and through the penis, passes through the middle of the prostate before passing through the penis. Sperms from the testes pass through a pair of small tubes, called the vas deferens. The vas deferens also passes through the sides of the prostate. Each vas deferens joins the urethra in the prostate gland, one on either side. The seminal vesicles are little pouches here, about 5 centimetres long, where prostate fluid and sperm mix and the mixture is stored before being discharged with sexual stimulation at the next ejaculation. The sperm from the testes does not become active for fertilisation until it has been mixed with fluid from the prostate gland. The prostate gland is therefore essential to maintain male fertility and ejaculation, even though it is not essential for male orgasm.

If the prostate gland is totally removed it is essential to create a new passage for the outflow of urine from the bladder. This is done by the surgeon joining the opening in the bladder to the passage (the urethra) in the base of the penis. During this operation the vas deferens on either side is tied off. Tying off, or ligation, of the vas deferens on either side as it passes through the groin region is also performed as a common form of male contraception known as a vasectomy.

2

What is cancer?

The word cancer is Latin for crab. The condition was called cancer in ancient times because an advanced cancer was compared with a crab having claws reaching out into surrounding tissues. A cancer, or malignant growth, is now known to be a continuous, purposeless, unwanted and uncontrolled growth of cells.

To understand the problems of prostate cancer it is important first to understand something about cancers in general. Hence throughout this book some description of cancers in general will be given before special reference is made to prostate cancer.

Most normal body tissues like the prostate are composed of cells that have the ability to divide and reproduce, but they do so only when there is a need. When this need has been satisfied they stop reproducing. Cells in some tissues, such as the skin or blood, wear out quickly and are constantly being replaced, but they are replaced only to meet the immediate need of the body; then reproduction of these cells stops. After injury, cells surrounding the injury site reproduce to replace and repair damaged tissues, but there is an inbuilt mechanism that stops the cell reproduction once the injury has been repaired and the wound has healed. There is a switch-off mechanism that stops cells dividing after healing is complete. However, in the case of a cancer the new cells are not needed, and cell reproduction continues for no good reason. Excessive numbers of abnormal cells are produced. There is no switching-off mechanism. The abnormal and unwanted cells accumulate in a lump and spread into surrounding tissues, causing damage and destruction. The excessive abnormal cancer cells also tend to invade blood vessels and lymph vessels, where they may travel to other parts of the body and establish new damaging colonies of unwanted growing cells. These colonies are called secondary or metastatic cancers.

A cancer is quite different from an infection. An infection is caused by germs or organisms from outside the body that invade body tissues and cause damage. The body defences recognise the invading germs as being composed of unwanted and damaging foreign invading material. The body defences thus establish protective measures to destroy these invading organisms. Invading cancer cells, on the other hand, are cells that have developed abnormally from the body's own cells. They are thus not recognised by the body's defences as foreign, so they continue to grow and invade without hindrance from the body's natural defences.

Although all malignant growths are commonly referred to as cancers, the word cancer (or carcinoma) is more correctly applied to a malignant growth of glandular cells or cells lining a hollow organ or a duct, or cells lining skin surfaces. For example, a cancer may start in cells lining the mouth, throat, stomach or bowel, cells lining the ducts of the breast or specialised breast glandular cells, cells lining the air passages in the lungs, or cells lining the cavity of the uterus or vagina, the kidney or bladder. Glandular cancers may develop in any gland. The prostate does have a small number of non-gland cells like fibrous cells, muscle cells and blood vessel cells in it, but most of the cells in the prostate are gland cells and these are the cells that have the greatest risk of growing into cancers.

How common is cancer?

Cancer occurs in all societies and in all parts of the world. It affects animals as well as people, and they develop similar cancers, including cancer of the prostate. In humans, cancer is known to have been present in ancient times, and it is still present in our modern age.

The risk of developing cancer is much less in young people than in older people, but cancer can affect people of any age, race or occupation, in any part of the world. However, the types of cancer most prevalent in a community vary with age, sex and race, as well as with the geography, the economic status, the environment and the habits of the people, including diet and tobacco smoking.

In Western societies cancer is responsible for about 20 per cent of deaths. Young people in Western societies are more at risk of dying as a result of accidents in homes or on the roads, but in older age groups of both sexes cancer is the leading cause of death. In most Western countries, including the UK, western Europe, the US, Canada, New Zealand and Australia, it has recently passed ischaemic heart disease (coronary artery disease) as the leading cause of death.

In men the prostate is the organ other than the skin that most commonly develops cancer, but not all prostate cancers develop to a degree that will cause problems during the man's natural lifetime. Some small prostate cancers remain in the prostate gland without causing any particular problems, and some will cause only minimal problems. These are known as 'latent cancers'. Others, described as invasive cancers, will grow more rapidly into other parts of the prostate gland where they may cause obstruction to the passage of urine, and still others (possibly one in four or five) will spread to other parts of the body. Those that do spread beyond the prostate spread especially to bones, where they cause serious trouble including pain and even fracture of the bones, and, eventually, death.

From the tables we can see that prostate cancer is the most common cancer of males in Western societies, although lung cancer causes more deaths. Prostate cancer is a cancer of older men and is uncommon before the age of 50. For women in Western societies breast cancer is both the most common cancer and the most common cause of cancer death (see tables 2.1 and 2.2). Lung cancer is the second most common cause of cancer death in women, and the numbers of women with lung cancer are still increasing because more women have taken up smoking in recent years. In fact the most recent figures from the US show that in that country lung cancer has become more common in women than breast cancer, and it is now clearly responsible for more cancer deaths than any other cancer in both sexes.

Table 2.1 The most common cancers in Western countries (other than common skin cancers)

Males	prostate
Females	breast
Both sexes together	large bowel (colon and rectum)

Table 2.2 The most common causes of cancer death in Western countries

Males	lung
Females	breast (now lung in the US)
Both sexes together	lung

Prostate cancer is still the most common cancer in men in Western countries (other than common skin cancers) but the numbers of men with prostate and lung cancer and women with breast cancer appear to have levelled off or to have even slightly decreased since about 1990. Breast cancer is about as common in women as invasive prostate cancer is in men, but the women affected by breast cancer are generally of a lower average age than the men affected by invasive prostate cancer.

Taking both sexes together, in most Western societies bowel cancer is the most common internal cancer. However, the cancer responsible for most deaths in the two sexes together is lung cancer, simply because in most cases it is diagnosed too late to be cured.

Benign tumours and malignant tumours

Benign enlargement of the prostate

Non-malignant (non-cancerous or benign) tumours are localised collections of cells that seem to be under some sort of control. They do not continue to grow and they do not spread. Benign tumours in glands are called adenomas. Although there is no apparent purpose in their growth, the cells look normal or almost normal, and once the clump of excessive cells reaches a certain size, it usually slows down or stops growing any further. All the cells of a benign tumour stay together as a lump or swelling that is usually surrounded by a capsule or lining of fibrous tissue.

Single adenomas are not often diagnosed in the prostate gland but the common generalised enlargement of all or part of the prostate gland, called hyperplasia, often begins by the age of 40 and is very common in older men. Although it affects older men of all societies and in all parts of the world, it is rather more common in Caucasian men (men of European ethnic origin) than in men of African or Asian descent who follow their traditional lifestyles in Africa or Asia.

Hyperplasia is caused by an increase in all the tissues that make up the prostate, including the muscular tissue, fibrous tissue and other non-gland tissue, not by disproportionate enlargement of the glandular part of the prostate. This enlargement (hyperplasia) may not cause any trouble at all, but in some men it may obstruct the flow of urine from the bladder to the penis. It is the most common cause of the difficulties in control and in passing urine that so often trouble older men. It is not a cancer, and as far as is known does not lead to cancer—cancers seem to be equally common in men with or without benign prostatic hyperplasia. Like benign tumours, hyperplasia of the prostate gland is due to excessive numbers of essentially normal-looking cells developing especially throughout the non-glandular tissue of the prostate gland. These cells have no tendency to spread into or to destroy other tissues.

If a doctor discovers a large, smooth prostate gland when using a gloved finger to carry out a digital rectal examination (DRE), the enlargement is more likely to be due to hyperplasia than to cancer.

Cancer of the prostate

With cancer or malignant growth, the doctor performing a rectal examination is likely to feel one or more hard or lumpy areas in the prostate. The prostate as a whole may or may not be enlarged.

When they are examined under a microscope the cells look abnormal and less like the cells from which they developed. As a rule, the more malignant the tumour the more abnormal the cells appear.

The multiplication of cells in the cancer continues without control, causing the tumour to get bigger and bigger. The tumour pushes into and grows into surrounding body tissues, damaging them. As the cancer grows and invades there is an increasing risk that it will grow into lymph vessels and blood vessels and other passages, and spread in the blood or lymph vessels to other parts of the body and establish secondary (metastatic) growths.

Secondary (metastatic) prostate cancer

'Secondary cancer' is a term used to describe a cancer that is growing in an organ or tissue some distance away from the tissue or organ in which it originally started. The most important differences between benign tumours and malignant tumours are that

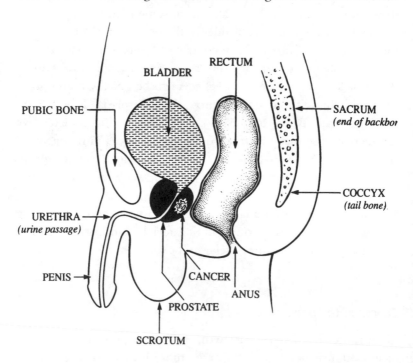

Figure 2.1 Diagram of the prostate gland with a cancer in its posterior aspect. The cancer can be felt by a doctor using a gloved finger to perform a digital examination of the rectum (DRE).

benign tumours tend to grow very slowly or not grow at all, and remain localised to the tissue in which they arose, whereas malignant tumours (cancers) tend to continue to grow and grow

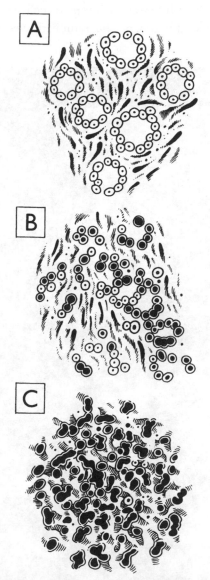

Figure 2.2 Illustrations of A: normal prostate gland cells, B: early or latent or non-invasive cancer cells, and C: aggressive, anaplastic, invasive cancer cells.

more rapidly, to grow into surrounding structures, damaging them, and to spread into tissues or organs away from the original or primary site of development.

To spread to distant sites, the malignant cells usually grow into blood vessels or lymph vessels. Clumps of cells break off and are carried by the bloodstream or the lymphatic vessels to a distant

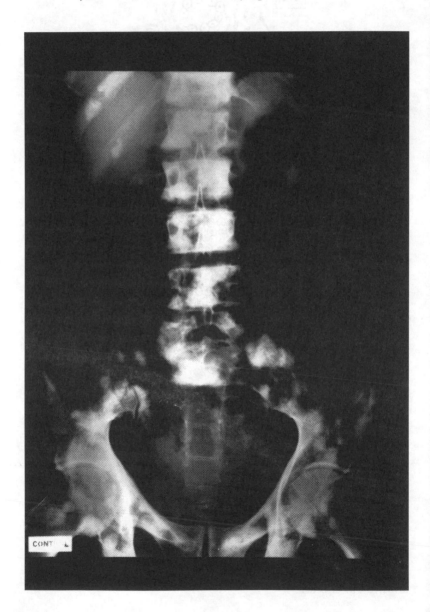

organ or tissue or to lymph nodes, where they may grow as secondary or metastatic tumours. The spreading cancer cells act something like 'seeds' being transported along blood or lymph vessels to a new 'soil' where they may take root and grow. In some cancers malignant cells may also spread along nerve sheaths or across body cavities such as the abdominal cavity, but this is not likely with prostate cancer.

The most common site for secondary spread of prostate cancers is via lymph vessels into lymph nodes. First, they grow in lymph nodes near the prostate gland, and then they spread into lymph nodes further away. In prostate cancer the next most common sites are spread by the bloodstream to bones, especially the bones of the pelvis, the lower vertebrae in the back (the backbone) or the long bone in the thigh, the femur. However, any bone can be affected, including any of the vertebrae, ribs, skull or bones in the limbs. Lymph nodes in the pelvis are also commonly involved and, at a later stage, lymph nodes in the abdomen and elsewhere.

The lungs, the liver or even the brain can also be involved in advanced cases. No tissue is exempt from developing a secondary,

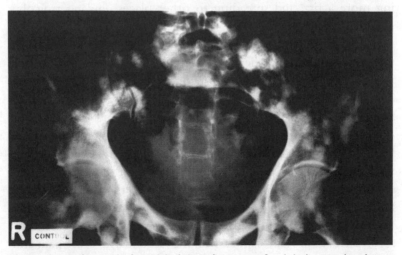

Figure 2.3 a (opposite) and b (above) X-rays of pelvic bones showing dark areas in bones where there is bone loss and bone destruction caused by metastatic cancer. The dense white or 'sclerotic' areas in the bones are due to calcium in many secondary deposits that are typical of prostate cancer secondaries in bones.

including the adrenal glands above the kidneys or the kidneys themselves. However, for no obvious reason, some organs and tissues tend to have a very low incidence of secondary growth. These include the spleen and muscles.

Is prostate cancer always dangerous?

If any cancer is detected early, while it is still small and before it has spread (metastasised) to another place, it can usually be completely removed surgically, or destroyed in some other way, so that its eradication or cure can be achieved before any serious damage has been done. If these early cancers are completely removed before they have spread, their danger will have been eliminated and the patient will be cured.

This is as true of prostate cancer as any other type of cancer. However, the majority of prostate cancers seem to grow very slowly or even to lie dormant as latent cancers, possibly for some years. Even if they do change into more aggressive invasive cancers they may still grow relatively slowly for some time before becoming more active and spreading to other places, endangering the patient's life.

Cancers are dangerous when they cause damage and destruction to surrounding tissues and when they spread to other organs and tissues where they establish secondary (or metastatic) cancers. The secondary growths damage and interfere with the function of and destroy the organ or tissue in which they are growing. For example, secondaries in the liver interfere with the function of the liver, and secondaries in the lung block air passages and interfere with breathing, leading to lung infection or pneumonia, and secondaries in the brain will cause pressure on the brain and interfere with brain function, often causing headaches first and possibly fits, convulsions or coma. Bones are the most common sites for secondaries of prostate cancer. In bones secondaries cause pain and weakness of the bones and in some cases the bones may collapse or break.

Fortunately most prostate cancers tend not to spread into other tissues during the natural life expectancy of the older men who have them. Most prostate cancers remain 'dormant' and relatively harmless for some months or years. These are sometimes called 'latent cancers', but even early invasive cancers may not be a threat to an elderly man with an otherwise limited life expectancy. In fact in only about one in four or five men who have a prostate cancer will this cancer cause his death; it is far more likely that one of the other 'natural causes' will take his life. He may live for years and die of another cause without ever being seriously troubled by his prostate cancer.

The big problem is that there is no way of knowing just which cancers will grow and spread rapidly and shorten a patient's life. Those that do grow and spread to other tissues cause a great deal of distress and often a miserable mode of death for the sufferer.

3

What causes cancer?

For generations doctors, researchers, philosophers and 'quacks' have been trying to find a single cause for all cancers, and consequently a single cure. No such single cause has been found and probably none exists.

Oncogenes

There are many different known factors that start changes in cells that lead to cancer. It is not known whether these causative factors all eventually act in the same way to activate a biological 'trigger' in the cell. Recent evidence suggests that they do not simply stimulate changes in cells that cause them to reproduce indiscriminately and so become a cancer. Instead, the cancer-causing factors possibly just weaken the body's natural defence mechanisms against cells that have a natural tendency to continue to reproduce. That is, rather than stimulating cells by applying an accelerator mechanism, it is possible that they interfere with the body's natural ability to apply a braking mechanism to cell growth. This braking mechanism appears to be at least partly an inbuilt suicide drive in cells that makes them self-destruct after they have served their useful period of life. This inbuilt self-destruction of cells when they are no longer needed is called *apoptosis*. A combination of these theories—both a stuck accelerator and faulty brakes—might be correct.

Many functions of our body cells are controlled by genes, coded in the DNA that makes up the chromosomes or genetic library of our cells. Like the genes that determine things like eye colour and hair colour and blood group, we inherit these controlling genes from our parents, and there is some evidence of a link between genetic make-up and some cancers.

All cells contain special genes called proto-oncogenes. These proto-oncogenes are responsible for switching on the self-limiting repair process when a tissue is injured or its cells are worn out and need to be replaced. When the repair is complete, the healing mechanism is switched off. The cancer-causing agents may cause the proto-oncogenes to change into oncogenes. Oncogenes can result from a number of factors including action of some viruses, action of chemical carcinogens, irradiation, and apparently spontaneous genetic mutation associated with ageing, or they might be inherited from a parent. The nature of the life-giving DNA of the cell is changed so that the switched-on mechanism of growth and repair continues instead of being switched off as it should be, and the cells that are produced do not undergo apoptosis.

There is evidence that some people have abnormal oncogenes in the inherited genetic make-up of their cells, and that in other people the inherited proto-oncogenes change into oncogenes due to other causes. These inherited abnormal proto-oncogenes or inherited oncogenes predispose those affected to a greater risk of cancer.

Other causes of cancer

Many common cancers can be traced to known causes or associated conditions. For example, exposure to ultraviolet light in sunshine is directly or indirectly responsible for most skin cancers. Tobacco causes cancers in many tissues—lungs, mouth, throat and larynx, as well as oesophagus, stomach, pancreas, kidney, bladder and even the breast. Viruses such as the papilloma virus are a direct cause of a few cancers, and others such hepatitis B, hepatitis C and the AIDS virus are indirect causes of others. Some cancers can be related to 'recreational' drugs—marijuana with lung cancer, and betel nut in the case of mouth cancer. Certain industrial carcinogens (such as excessive soot, asbestos, benzene, aniline dyes, phosphorus, arsenic, and some wood and metal chippings), some air pollutants, and some forms of irradiation (excessive exposure to X-rays as was common when they were first used, and exposure to radiation from atomic bombs) have been incriminated in other cancers. However, no one of these, nor any other specific cause, has yet been incriminated in causing prostate cancer.

For a lot of cancers the cancer might have developed from a pre-existing benign tumour or other pre-existing benign abnormality. It was believed for a long time that pre-existing prostatic hyperplasia might have been a precursor of prostate cancer, but recent studies have found no convincing evidence to support this. Both prostatic hyperplasia and prostate cancer are common in older men of Western societies, so both conditions are commonly present in the same patient. Men with and without evidence of benign prostatic hyperplasia seem to be about equally prone to developing prostate cancer. In fact in Asian countries prostate hyperplasia is a rather common condition in older men, although not quite as common as it is in Western countries, but clinical invasive prostate cancer is relatively uncommon in Asian countries.

Of the causes and associations mentioned above, the closest known association with common cancers is with tobacco smoking, but there is no convincing evidence that tobacco smoking causes prostate cancer. Non-smokers appear to be just as prone to getting prostate cancer as are smokers. However, there is one important difference between smokers and non-smokers. Prostate cancer in smokers tends to grow and spread more aggressively than in non-smokers. So, although prostate cancer appears to be no more common in smokers, smokers develop a more lethal form of the disease.

It was once believed that the birth control procedure known as vasectomy increased the risk of prostate cancer, but recent studies have not found any association between vasectomy and prostate cancer—neither an increase nor a decrease.

History of a previous cancer

People who have been cured of one cancer often ask about the risk of developing a second cancer of a different type. Although it is true that some people have an increased predisposition towards developing cancer, in most cases the risk of developing a second serious cancer is not great. There is no evidence that men who have previously been treated for another cancer have any greater or lesser risk of subsequently getting cancer of the prostate.

Is cancer contagious?

There is no evidence that in the normal course of events cancer can be passed from one individual to another.

AIDS (acquired immune deficiency syndrome) is caused by a virus infection that may predispose infected people to cancer due to damage to natural immune defences. AIDS patients have lowered resistance to infections and are more prone than non-infected people to some forms of cancer, but there is no particular association with prostate cancer.

Liver cancer is not infectious, but a common cause of liver cancer is infection by the hepatitis B or hepatitis C viruses. These hepatitis infections do spread easily from person to person, mainly via food or intimate contact, so liver cancer develops more commonly in people who have been infected, but there is no evidence of any relationship between prostate cancer and any hepatitis infection.

The human papilloma virus (HPV) can be transmitted sexually, and infection with the virus can cause cancer of the cervix, vagina or vulva in women and cancer of the penis in men, but no association between infection with the human papilloma virus and prostate cancer has been seen.

Is there an inherited risk?

In some relatively uncommon cancers there is a strong hereditary factor; in other cancers there is a less obvious slight hereditary factor. For most cancers, however, there is no evidence of any hereditary factor at all.

Among the cancers with a strong hereditary factor is a condition called familial polyposis coli, in which half the children of an affected parent are likely to develop the condition of multiple polyps (tumours projecting on a stalk) in the mucous membrane lining the large bowel. A particular gene inherited from one or other parent is responsible for transmission of this abnormality, which will cause affected people to develop cancer in the bowel, usually by the age of 40 years.

The more common cancers that show an increased familial incidence include cancers of the breast, stomach and bowel. Although in most families the increased risk of cancer in relatives of sufferers is small, in occasional families there may be a considerably increased risk. For example, there have been rare reports of families in which about half the female blood relatives have developed breast cancer. What is responsible for this apparent increased risk in some families is uncertain. It may be strictly an inherited oncogene that affects the cells, tissues, or body defences, or it may be that members of these families are more likely to have similar habits or be affected by other similar living conditions (environment). It might also be due to a combination of these factors.

Prostate cancer is more common in some families than others, but it is not yet clear what is most responsible. Studies are presently being made to determine whether an inherited gene (an oncogene) is responsible. If invasive prostate cancer does develop in men younger than 60, the risk of such a cancer occurring in their male relatives is increased four times. These male relatives should therefore be kept under regular observation.

Although a genetic factor does appear to be associated with prostate cancers in younger men (men younger than 60), such cases of early onset of prostate cancer are relatively uncommon. For the majority of patients with prostate cancer other factors appear to be more significant, especially age but also probably diet.

What about age?

In general, the risk of developing most cancers increases with age. There is no more obvious association between increasing age and cancer than in the case of cancer of the prostate. This cancer is uncommon before the age of 50 but thereafter the incidence increases with age. Studies have shown that in Western societies possibly 15–20 per cent of men at the age of 50 will have cells that have some features of early malignant cells in their prostate gland, but by 90 years of age more than 80 per cent of men will have some prostate cells that appear to be malignant.

In men in Western societies, prostate cancer is now the most common cancer, other than the common small skin cancers, and it is especially common in men over the age of 65 years.

Does race play a part?

Some cancers are more prevalent in people of some races than in other races. Whether the significant factor is a genetic or racial factor, or whether it is more likely to be due to environment, habits, diet or other influences, such as the general health and age of the people, is hard to determine.

Examples of increased racial or ethnic incidence of certain cancers include the higher incidence of stomach cancer in Japan and Korea and to a lesser extent in Scandinavia, the Netherlands and the former Czechoslovakia; the high incidence of cancer of the oesophagus in certain African tribes including the Bantu in South Africa but not in the white population; the high incidence of liver cancer (hepatoma) in Malaysians, other South-East Asians and Africans; the high incidence of cancer of the post-nasal space in ethnic Chinese, especially people from Kwantung province, and even in their descendants born outside China; and the high incidence of both breast cancer and prostate cancer, as well as cancer of the large bowel, in Europeans and people of European descent. In Israel, a country with one of the highest incidences of thyroid cancer, the disease is more common amongst Jews born in Europe than in those born in Asia. In South Africa, Bantus have a much higher incidence of thyroid cancer than do blacks from other regions.

It seems that, while there are genetic influences that predispose people of different races to develop different cancers, it is hard to know with any particular cancer whether the most significant factors are genetic or due to social habits or diet or result from economic or other influences, or if they result from a combination of a number of different factors. For example, there is a high incidence of melanoma and other skin cancers in people of northern European descent who live in tropical and sub-tropical climates, and this is known to be due to the genetic factor of fair skin plus the environmental factor of exposure to strong sunshine.

The incidence of prostate cancer in Western societies increased during the twentieth century. It has remained much lower in Asians and Africans who have continued to live in their traditional lifestyles in Asia and Africa. Those men of Asian or African ethnic background who have adopted Western lifestyles in Western countries have an increased incidence of prostate cancer similar to that of their fellow citizens of Caucasian ethnic backgrounds. In fact post-mortem studies have shown a similar incidence of latent cancer in all races studied. It seems therefore that some lifestyle or environmental factor is of greater significance than race in the risk of developing prostate cancer. However, the picture is not simple. Although Africans in Africa have a significantly lower risk of developing prostate cancer than have Caucasians in the West, prostate cancer is significantly more common and more aggressive in African Americans than in white Americans.

Geography and environment

Although the incidence of a particular type of cancer varies from country to country and even varies within the one country according to geographic conditions, it is often difficult to be sure whether the difference is essentially due to different geographic or climatic elements, or to race, social habits or other environmental differences, or possibly to combinations of these.

The association of skin cancer and melanoma with fair-skinned people living in a sunny climate is obvious. The incidence is highest in fair-skinned people living in sunny climates in Australia and in the sunny southern parts of the United States.

The association between the high incidence of prostate cancer in the UK, Europe, North America, Australia and New Zealand and much lower incidence in India, China, Japan and other Asian and in African countries appears not to be related to race or geography nearly as much as to diets or other lifestyle practices. If people from Asian or African countries move to Western countries or adopt Western diets and lifestyle practices, their risk of prostate cancer becomes similar to that of Western men of European ethnic origin.

Occupation

There is no convincing evidence of any significant association between occupation and prostate cancer.

Smoking

The most obvious and widespread carcinogen in present-day society is tobacco. The habit of smoking outweighs all other known influences as a cause of many types of serious cancers in present-day men and women. The incidence of lung cancer is increased some eight to ten times in smokers when compared with non-smokers, and the risk is directly related to the amount of tobacco smoked and inhaled.

Smoking tobacco has not been found to increase the incidence of prostate cancer. However, as mentioned previously, it does appear to be responsible for causing prostate cancers to become more aggressive in smokers.

Alcohol

Heavy alcohol drinkers have an increased incidence of cancer of the mouth and throat, oesophagus, stomach, liver and pancreas, but there is no evidence to associate heavy alcohol consumption with prostate cancer.

Previous sexual behaviour

Some men are concerned that their previous sexual behaviour might be related to their risk of prostate cancer. They worry that they might have avoided prostate cancer if their previous sexual lifestyle had been different.

Some studies have been made, but there is no evidence that multiple sexual partners, heterosexual or homosexual practices, masturbation, celibacy, or any other variation of sexual behaviour has any association with either an increased or a decreased risk of prostate cancer. Although there are many 'old men's tales' about sexual activity and prostate cancer, this is at least one area where the basis for such tales remains a mystery, more likely related to puritanical thinking than to scientific fact.

Cultural and social customs

Cultural and social customs may have a relationship with development of some cancers, but apart from an apparent association with diet there is no evidence for any other significant association with prostate cancer.

Members of the Seventh Day Adventist Church have a lower incidence of many cancers than do other members of Western communities. This appears to be associated with a number of lifestyle factors, including their high-fibre vegetarian diet, abstention from smoking and alcohol, and their strictly monogamous sexual behaviour. A reduced incidence of prostate cancer has been reported in those Church members who practise strict vegetarianism with no intake of animal products, not even eggs or dairy products.

The best clues about causes

Apart from the cellular degeneration and replacement associated with increasing age, the closest apparent associations with prostate cancer are possibly familial, possibly racial and possibly geographic, as mentioned above, but the association most likely to be of significance is related to diet.

Diets

There is an association between diet and some cancers of the digestive tract. Certainly a high-fibre diet appears to be protective against bowel cancer. The different incidences of other cancers, especially differences in the incidence of breast and prostate cancers between people in Asia and Caucasians (people of European ethnic origin), may also be related to diet.

Traditionally, Asian peoples have a diet with a high content of legumes (peas, lentils, soya beans etc.). Legumes have greater amounts of the naturally occurring plant hormones known as isoflavones than any other plant species. These are the most concentrated and most active of the plant oestrogens (phytoestrogens). Studies suggest that this may be a factor in the relatively low incidence of breast diseases (including cancer) in Asian women and the relatively low incidence of prostate cancer in Asian males. There is evidence that before Europeans changed their diets from one high in legumes and other plant foods to one high in animal products with the industrial revolution about a hundred or two hundred years ago, the incidence of breast and prostate diseases, including cancer, in Europeans was lower than it is at present.

Members of the Seventh Day Adventist Church have a lower than average incidence of most cancers, including prostate and breast cancer but also cancers of the oesophagus, stomach, pancreas, colon and rectum. However, as well as being vegetarians with a high fibre intake and low meat and animal fat consumption, Church members are usually non-smokers and do not drink alcohol. Such differences in lifestyle may well be more significant. A study of male members of the Seventh Day Adventist Church found that those Church members whose diet included meat, eggs, cheese and milk had a greater incidence of prostate cancer than those who refrained from all animal products.

For cancers other than prostate, breast, bowel and possibly pancreas, there is no evidence that these particular dietary factors—legumes and fibre—play a part, although other dietary factors may play a part in stomach, oesophagus and liver cancer.

There are so many variable factors among people of different population groups that it is always difficult to prove which particular factor or factors might be responsible for any difference in the incidence of cancer. For example, as well as differences in diet there may be genetic differences, racial differences, environmental differences, or differences in social habits or customs such as smoking, differences in the incidence of parasites or infections, or even in occupational stress or psychological factors.

The evidence of association between diet and cancer is strongest for cancer of the large bowel but it is also increasingly apparent in both breast cancer in women and prostate cancer in men. Dietary studies are now being undertaken to measure the effect of the naturally occurring plant hormones (the isoflavone type of phytoestrogens) in leguminous plants like soya beans. These studies should decide if diet or some other factor is the reason that people in Asian countries, where there is a high intake of these foods, have a lower incidence of a number of problems, including prostate cancer, that are common in Western societies where the intake of isoflavones is low. Laboratory studies and clinical studies have confirmed that prostate cancer cells appear to become less dangerous after exposure to preparations made from isoflavones or when a patient with a typical Western diet takes increased quantities of these plant hormones by mouth.

Psychological or emotional associations

Amongst the more unusual theories for causes of cancer has been a suggestion that, like emotional and some mental (psychosomatic) illnesses, cancer may result from an unnatural suppression of the 'fight or flight' response to anxiety or stress. It has been suggested that if a stressful situation persists over a long period and the person concerned feels that whatever action he or she takes will be wrong, a subconscious decision to escape through death by cancer may result.

There is little evidence to support such a theory, although some retrospective studies have indicated that a high proportion of cancer patients have experienced some form of severe stress in the period six months to two years before the onset of illness. Whether this incidence of stress is different in people who have not developed cancer is not yet certain.

Most psychologists would not claim that psychological reactions are a direct cause of cancer, but some feel that they may play a part alongside known chemical, genetic, environmental, dietary, degenerative, viral or radiation causes. Certainly, the association of possible psychological factors in people given a diagnosis of cancer has confirmed a need for additional psychological support for many patients. Such support may be best given by psychiatrists, clinical psychologists, social workers or other specially trained health workers. For some patients the help of an understanding member of the clergy or other spiritual adviser can be most helpful.

For any patient with cancer, the possible association with psychological factors and the need for psychological adjustment has been given by a variety of alternative or fringe medicine practitioners as a reason for their treatment by faith healing, meditation and even, in some cases, for a variety of herbal or other potions.

For men with prostate cancer these possible psychological associations are generally less obvious. This is probably because the group of people affected is generally older and because of the traditional reluctance of men to admit to emotional disturbance, but also because the progression of the disease is often slower than is common in most other cancers.

4

Can prostate cancer be prevented?

Unfortunately, there is no known way of making any individual immune to the development of any cancer. However, the risk of many cancers can be considerably reduced by taking certain precautions and avoiding cancer-causing (carcinogenic) influences.

The greatest hope for being able to reduce the risk of development of prostate cancer appears to be to learn some lessons from the dietary practices of those ethnic groups, communities or countries with a low incidence of prostate cancer.

Smoking

The most obvious preventive measure in reducing the risk of developing many serious cancers is to avoid smoking.

As far as prostate cancer is concerned, it appears that smokers and non-smokers have a similar risk of getting this cancer, but the outlook is better for those men who are not smokers. Either their cancers are generally less aggressive, or the body's natural defences against cancer are stronger in non-smokers.

Diet and dietary supplements

Studies are presently being conducted to determine whether diet can change the incidence of prostate cancer.

There is a lot of circumstantial evidence to indicate that men who adhere to a vegetarian diet will have a reduced risk of prostate cancer. There are two main theoretical reasons for this. First is the high content of plant hormones in vegetarian diets, especially the isoflavone types of phytoestrogens and related compounds. These are particularly plentiful in peas, beans and other legumes, especially soy, and may be responsible for the low incidence of prostate cancer in Asians, Africans and men of other 'less developed' countries whose diets consist predominantly of plant foods. Another hypothesis is that the absence of animal fats may well be a significant factor in contributing to the low incidence of prostate cancer in vegetarians. There is also evidence to support this proposal.

A further, as yet unproven but widely held, belief is that diets with relatively high levels of the anti-oxidant vitamins A, C and E, and certain trace elements, especially selenium, might have some protective value against cancer. This causes some nutritionists to recommend addition of these supplements to the daily intake of Westerners. Although still unproven, some supplements of these anti-oxidant vitamins and selenium might be of some protective value, provided they are well measured and not taken in toxic amounts. Vitamin A and selenium, especially, can be toxic if too much is taken.

Recent dietary studies, especially from Harvard medical school in the US and from Israel, suggest that *lycopene*, the substance that gives tomatoes their red colour, may give some protection against certain cancers. Laboratory studies, as well as studies of both humans and animals, suggest that lycopene may protect against a number of degenerative diseases, including heart disease, degeneration of the eye, and some cancers, including prostate cancer. Until more studies have been completed we can only conclude that these results reinforce the value of certain natural foods in the diet, including tomatoes and tomato products. It also appears that lycopene is better absorbed from cooked tomatoes or tomato paste than from fresh raw tomatoes or tomato juice; it can now also be produced in commercial quantities from especially genetically engineered tomatoes as well as some other fruits.

All legumes—including peas, beans and especially soy— contain relatively large quantities of the plant hormones (phyto- estrogens) called isoflavones. Red clover is a legume, and the most active isoflavones are found in it in much greater concentration than in any other known plant source, including soy. Tablets are now available that contain in one tablet as much of the isoflavones as is consumed in a traditional Asian daily diet. An Australian-produced red clover product, marketed as Trinovin, is designed specifically for this purpose and contains at least as much of the most active phytoestrogens than are present in a traditional Asian daily diet and an even broader range of them. Studies are presently being conducted to determine whether by taking just one of these tablets daily the risk of prostate cancer can be reduced in men who otherwise have a traditional Western diet.

It appears that the risk of developing prostate cancer could be reduced for Western men if they adopted a completely vegetarian diet with a high soy content including the use of soy milk. This suggestion is unlikely to be adhered to by most Westerners, and is possibly no more beneficial than taking one small isoflavone tablet daily in conjunction with a diet with reduced levels of animal fat. I believe that it would be more logical to reduce the intake of animal products, especially animal fat in meat and dairy products, and in addition to this modified Western diet to take one concentrated isoflavone tablet daily.

5

Symptoms of prostate cancer

Symptoms are the signs that a person notices as being wrong and cause the person to seek medical attention.

Symptoms of cancer may result from two effects. The first is the local effect of the cancer itself. The second is the more general effect of the cancer on the person as a whole. The earlier a patient seeks medical attention for anything unusual or different, the more likely it will be that any cancer will be detected at a curable stage.

Prostate cancer can be present in some men, possibly for some years, without causing any symptoms. Usually local features are noticed first. The common symptoms of both prostate cancer and benign prostatic hyperplasia are various types of difficulty in passing urine. The flow may be slow to start and slow to stop, and there may be incontinence (that is, uncontrolled dribbling of urine), frequency of wanting to pass urine, possibly including several times at night, or sometimes pain on passing urine. Occasionally there can be complete obstruction to the passage of urine, a very painful and unpleasant experience needing urgent medical attention.

These symptoms result from obstruction to the passage of urine resulting from the prostate pressing on the urethra, the passage for urine to pass from the bladder through the prostate and penis (see figure 1.1, chapter 1). The most common cause for these difficulties is benign enlargement of the prostate due to prostate hyperplasia, but cancer is the next most common cause.

Sometimes benign prostatic hyperplasia and cancer are both present, as both conditions become more common in men with increasing age.

The main general effects of prostate cancer are usually due to the cancer having spread from the prostate to other tissues or organs. Bone is the most common site of spread, and secondary (metastatic) growths damage or destroy local areas of bone. Affected bone may be painful. The bones most commonly affected are vertebrae in the back, bones of the pelvis, and the large thigh bone called the femur, but any bone, including ribs, skull or bones in the limbs, can be affected. In X-rays, secondaries of prostate cancer usually show as round white areas in the bones due to their increased content of calcium (see figure 2.3). Sometimes a spontaneous fracture of an affected bone can be the first indication of a prostate cancer.

Rarely the first evidence of a prostate cancer, as with other cancers, can be general symptoms such as malaise, lassitude and loss of energy, loss of appetite, weight loss, or the effects of anaemia. The effects of the spread of secondaries to other organs such as lungs or liver are very rarely the first indication of prostate cancer.

Screening tests

The PSA test

There is no single absolutely reliable screening test to diagnose the presence of prostate cancer. However, the PSA (prostate specific antigen) blood test is a test commonly used to detect the presence of some sort of abnormality in the prostate. Prostate specific antigens are enzymes produced by prostate gland cells, and their level in the circulation is measured by the PSA blood test. When the number of prostate gland cells is increased or there is increased activity in the prostate gland, the level of PSA in the blood is usually raised. The abnormality causing a raised PSA might be any of inflammation or hyperplasia or cancer. An elevated PSA index is often the first indication of the presence of a prostate cancer, but not all men with prostate cancer have a raised PSA.

PSA levels in blood are measured in 'units' of one microgram per litre of blood. This has been found to be a very convenient measurement. The normal upper limit of PSA in men up to about the age of 50 is 2.5. As the prostate usually slowly becomes a little larger with increasing age and there are thus more prostate cells producing PSA, the upper limit of normal by the age of 60 is about 3.5. In men of 80 a PSA up to 10 may be considered normal.

At this stage the test is the best simple screening indicator, but it is not totally reliable. The level can sometimes be raised in conditions other than cancer, and it can occasionally be normal when prostate cancer is present. If the PSA used as a screening test finds the PSA index raised above 4 units in men of 55 or 60 years of age, it suggests there is an abnormality in the prostate gland. Although an index of between 4 and 10 is most commonly due to benign hyperplasia, the higher the index the more likely it is due to cancer. An index greater than 10, especially if it is rising in successive tests, is usually an indication of cancer, even though the patient may have no symptoms of the disease.

In the past the most common and useful screening test for prostate cancer was a digital rectal examination (DRE) (see below). A hard or lumpy prostate was regarded as the most useful indication of a possible prostate cancer. In recent years it has been common for family doctors and specialists to have a PSA test carried out as an initial cancer screening test in men over 50 years of age. This, together with a digital rectal examination of the prostate (DRE), has been an increasingly common practice, especially in the USA.

The PSA is the simplest and least disturbing prostate test for men concerned about the possibility of having a prostate cancer. While there is some controversy as to whether PSA testing should be used as a screening test, most doctors agree that it is valuable in the general follow-up tests for men who have had surgery to remove the entire prostate gland (prostatectomy). If prostatectomy has successfully removed all prostate tissue, including all prostate cancer cells, the PSA should fall to virtually zero. If the PSA falls but later starts to rise again, it is strong evidence that the cancer has recurred in some part of the man's body.

Although a significantly raised PSA does not necessarily mean that cancer is present, it does suggest the need for further investigation. This may include ultrasound and biopsy of the prostate gland. Some doctors advise a PSA as a screening test every two years or so in men over 50 or in younger men with a strong family history of prostate cancer, just as a mammogram is recommended as a screening test every two years or so for women at risk of breast cancer. Other doctors do not recommend such regular testing, or indeed any testing at all. This is because even if cancer is detected, what best to do about it is often controversial. In contrast to screening for breast cancer, where there is now clear evidence that screening leading to early treatment does improve the life expectancy of women whose breast cancer is detected, there is as yet no proof that PSA screening for prostate cancer does significantly improve the prognosis or outlook for men with prostate cancer.

This issue is presently most controversial, and is discussed further on pages 81–6. Worldwide, experts are divided as to whether to carry out routine PSA testing or not to test in any man without prostate symptoms. That is, they disagree on whether they should risk ringing alarm bells when it is still uncertain what they mean or what is the best thing to do about the problem if an alarm does ring.

Digital rectal examination (DRE)

A digital rectal examination or DRE is carried out with the patient lying on his side with his legs curled up in the foetal position. The doctor wears a rubber glove and covers the index finger with a gentle lubricant, like baby oil, and gently inserts the index finger through the anus to feel the prostate gland in front and other contents of the rectum and in the pelvis as far as the finger will reach. If a lump is felt in the prostate gland it can sometimes alert the doctor to the presence of a cancer while the cancer is still small.

The examination usually takes less than a minute but can give the doctor a lot of useful information. The examination may be a little unpleasant but it is not painful and no anaesthetic is required. Although it may feel a little embarrassing for the patient, he should remember that most people have had such an examination at some time, especially women who have had babies, and every doctor, male and female, has carried out this sort of examination many times.

A digital examination of the prostate is generally recommended as part of a general annual health check for men over 50, along with such tests as blood cholesterol and a urine test for sugar. In a rectal examination, not only is the size, shape and consistency of the prostate noted, but the rectum and pelvis are also examined for any other possible abnormality, such as bleeding or even a cancer in the rectum.

Digital rectal examinations (DRE) were formerly referred to as PR (per rectum) examinations.

Ultrasound

Ultrasound cannot by itself diagnose prostate cancer. While most doctors consider that a regular two-yearly ultrasound study is taking screening testing too far, it is being done in some clinics, especially in the US. Regular ultrasound testing would seem to be more appropriate if it is confined to men at special risk, such as men with a strong family history of prostate cancer or men with a persistently raised PSA, especially if the PSA continues to rise.

In an ultrasound test, a thin tube is inserted through the anus into the rectum. An ultrasound probe in the tube allows ultrasound images of the prostate gland to be seen on a television screen and recorded on paper.

If a shadow indicating a lump is seen in the ultrasound image, a small sample of prostate tissue can be taken for examination (biopsied), using a spring-loaded biopsy punch (see chapter 7). Again this is painless but a little uncomfortable. The biopsy can be taken only if the patient is well prepared, with a clean empty rectum and antibiotic cover; if not, a separate biopsy date will be arranged.

After 20 minutes or so the test is all complete, apart from the microscopic examination of tissue if a biopsy was taken. The patient should feel no ill effects from a simple ultrasound examination and should be able to go home or return to work or whatever he has to do.

While annual PSA testing of a blood sample and annual digital rectal examination of the prostate are commonly accepted as screening tests, in most clinics and in most countries the ultrasound is usually reserved as a diagnostic test when an abnormality has already been detected by PSA or digital examination.

The value of precautionary screening

As will be discussed later, there is a great deal of controversy as to whether any screening tests for prostate cancer can be justified in men at risk but with no symptoms. Even if evidence of an early cancer is detected, as yet there is no certain way of knowing whether or not this cancer has the potential to grow and spread and be a threat to the patient's life during the term of his natural life expectancy. In other words, in any particular case there is no way of knowing whether the cancer should be treated or not, taking into consideration the likely complications of prostate surgery or any other treatment, and the significant possibility that the cancer may not be one that will progress sufficiently to cause symptoms during the patient's expected lifetime.

Considering a diagnosis

Differential diagnosis

Depending on symptoms and other evidence of a health problem, the diagnosis of cancer must be certain before any plan of cancer treatment can be recommended. The doctor may well suspect cancer, but proper consideration must be given to other possible prostate problems or other health problems that could be responsible for any patient's symptoms. These are at least listed and considered in the doctor's mind. Such a list is called the 'differential diagnosis'.

The symptoms most likely to be associated with prostate cancer are related to partial or occasionally complete obstruction of the flow of urine. The man may have dribbling, frequency, difficulty in starting, or incomplete finishing of flow of urine. He may get out of bed frequently at night to pass urine, or he may have to squeeze hard to get the urine to flow. Occasionally a man may first complain of complete blockage to the flow of urine—a very painful and distressing experience requiring urgent medical help.

Each of these symptoms is more commonly caused by prostate hyperplasia (non-cancerous enlargement of the prostate), but they can be caused by a prostate cancer. Prostate hyperplasia must therefore be high on the differential diagnosis list; that is, the doctor must be sure that prostate hyperplasia is not the cause of the problems.

In recent years, one of the most common features leading a doctor to consider a diagnosis of prostate cancer has been the finding of a raised PSA level. This may show up when the doctor has examined a patient for an unrelated condition or when a PSA has been arranged as a screening procedure in a man who may not have any relevant symptoms. Among the well-known reasons for an elevated PSA, other than cancer, are prostate hyperplasia and acute or chronic inflammation of the prostate arising from a recent or long-standing infection (prostatitis).

With a raised PSA, therefore, both hyperplasia and prostatitis must be added to the differential diagnosis list. The doctor must consider both these possibilities. The PSA levels may be raised in men with prostate hyperplasia and no cancer, but PSA levels that continue to rise and reach high levels, 12 or 16 or more, are likely to indicate prostate cancer.

Occasionally the first real evidence of a prostate cancer is the presence of a secondary cancer in one or more bones. This may show up as bone pain, a spontaneous fracture of a bone, or a bone defect seen in an X-ray taken for some other condition. If such troubles occur in bones the possibility of prostate cancer being the cause must be considered.

On rare occasions a prostate cancer may first cause symptoms when it spreads (metastasises) to lungs, liver or brain. Sometimes these secondary cancers can be in bones in the back or pelvis, causing pressure on the spinal cord or pressure on a major nerve, with severe pain passing down a leg or threatening to cause paralysis. In all of these situations the possibility that prostate cancer is responsible must also be considered, just as it will have to be considered when the general health of an elderly man deteriorates, possibly with weight loss, anaemia or just general debility.

Of all these possibilities, benign prostate hyperplasia is the most common cause of problems that are most likely to be confused with prostate cancer. Hyperplasia is commonly the only prostate problem present, although it may be present in a man who also has prostate cancer. The doctor will be aware of the possibility of both conditions being present.

Prostate hyperplasia

Cancer of the prostate is uncommon before the age of 50, but in Western countries it is the most common cancer, other than skin cancers, in men over the age of 65. It became increasingly common in Western countries during the twentieth century. Prostate hyperplasia is also very common in older men in virtually all races and societies. Some prostate enlargement seems to develop from the age of 40 onwards, but only when it becomes excessive, particularly in prostate tissue around the urethra (the passage for urine to pass through the prostate), is it likely to cause symptoms related to difficulty, frequency or hesitancy in passing urine. It is not uncommon for both conditions to be present in the one person at the same time.

Although both hyperplasia and prostate cancer are common, hyperplasia is more common than cancer. It is more common to find hyperplasia without cancer than to find cancer without hyperplasia.

The prostate enlargement related to hyperplasia is composed of all the types of tissue found in the prostate gland. There is increased muscle and supporting fibrous tissue around the increased numbers of prostate gland cells. There is more and irregular glandular tissue composed of muscle fibres, fibrous tissue strands and often distorted patterns of essentially normal-looking gland cells. Otherwise the gland cells do not show the features of the abnormality seen in cancer (see figure 2.2).

Hyperplasia alone, without cancer, usually causes a uniform enlargement of the prostate on one or other or both sides. To the doctor performing a digital rectal examination, the enlargement feels normal in consistency (it is softish and rubbery), with a smooth groove felt between the two sides (or two lobes) of the gland. A hard nodule or lump in the prostate, or generalised hardness or lumpiness, is unlikely to be caused by hyperplasia alone. Occasionally it may be due to a previous infection in the prostate (prostatitis), possibly from a urinary infection or a sexually transmitted infection earlier in life. Occasionally calcified lumps like small stones may be present in the prostate as a consequence of a low-grade or minor infection in previous years. If a low-grade infection or subsequent low-grade inflammation is still present, the prostate might still be somewhat tender.

Ultrasound is very helpful in showing the presence or absence of nodules in the prostate even if they could not be felt with the examining doctor's finger. Ultrasound will also show just where in the prostate the lumps are, their size, and their number. If the lumps are calcified, which is more likely to be a result of a previous infection than cancer, the ultrasound will help to show this. However, ultrasound does not show what kind of cells are present in any lump, and therefore ultrasound alone cannot diagnose cancer.

Pathology diagnosis

The final diagnosis can be made only by taking a piece of the abnormal tissue (a biopsy) and having the tissue sample prepared and examined microscopically by an expert pathologist. The pathologist can see whether cancer cells are present and from their appearance can tell whether they appear to be aggressive cancer cells or low-grade cancer cells. If aggressive cancer cells are found and they are seen to be invading into nearby prostate tissues, it can be assumed that this is a dangerous form of cancer. If, however, the pathologist finds only minor changes in the cells and they appear not to have moved from where they were expected to be, this is classed as a latent cancer (see figure 2.2).

There is as yet no way of knowing for sure whether a latent cancer will become aggressive and be a danger to the owner's life, or whether it might remain unchanged or virtually unchanged during the patient's otherwise expected lifetime.

6

Treatment of hyperplasia without cancer

Traditional surgical treatment: TURP

Until fairly recently the only really effective treatment of prostate hyperplasia was by surgery. The position of the prostate, deep in the pelvis and surrounded by other vital structures (see chapter 1), makes this difficult, so before the current surgical techniques of trans-urethral resection of the prostate (TURP) were developed prostate surgery was gruesome and carried considerable risk.

In the nineteenth century, men with severe obstruction to flow of urine either had to learn to pass a tube (catheter) up through their own penis and along their urethra to the bladder, or were sometimes subjected to an operation in which an opening was made in the bladder through the lower abdominal wall for urine to drain out. The stories of the gentry carrying a catheter in their top hats were sometimes true. With irritating rubber catheters in those pre-antibiotic days, infection of the bladder, kidneys and the urethra was rife, and so men who needed to use a catheter usually did not survive for very long.

In the first half of the twentieth century, the standard treatment for prostate hyperplasia (or indeed for prostate cancer) that was causing severe urinary obstructive symptoms was removal of the whole prostate by surgery. This was a bloody operation needing prolonged hospital care, often treatment of severe and prolonged blood loss, and a catheter to be in place for an extended period, possibly for some weeks, after the operation.

During this period the first instruments were designed to cut away the obstructing prostate tissue with a sharp cutting blade at the end of the long thin metal instrument (the resectoscope) passed up through the penis, where the urethra allows the resectoscope an easy passage. This was a distinct improvement in most cases, as it meant the surgeon did not have to work around the other organs in the crowded lower abdomen, but blood loss after the operation was still a major problem.

The next major improvement was a similar technique with the surgeon being able to cut away obstructing prostate tissue using a diathermy loop instead of a blade on the end of the resectoscope. The diathermy loop is a small loop of fine wire that is heated when the surgeon switches on an electrical current. The tissue is removed by a cutting and burning process that seals the small blood vessels at the same time. Better resectoscopes are now used that give the surgeon a good view of the whole process via a system of mirrors and lenses.

This operation is now safe and effective in removing the right amount of prostate tissue with a minimal amount of blood loss. TURP is commonly carried out under a spinal anaesthetic but sometimes a general anaesthetic is used. With a spinal anaesthetic the patient may be awake or sleeping or only lightly anaesthetised during the procedure.

The most common problem immediately after a TURP operation is still bleeding. A plastic non-irritating catheter through the penis to the bladder must be left in for a few days, to ensure that urine passes freely and to see and allow control of the inevitable small amount of bleeding that will follow. The nursing and medical staff carefully measure the amount of urine passed and watch to be sure that the amount of blood in the urine gets less each day and eventually stops.

Nowadays blood transfusion is rarely required after a TURP operation, but the surgical team must be prepared to give a transfusion if there is continued blood loss. Pain-relieving medications are usually required for a few days post-operatively. As a catheter may be needed, usually for only one or two days but possibly for a week or so after the operation, the risk of infection is consider-able, and antibiotics are given to cover this risk.

Longer-term problems

In the longer term there may be one or more of four main problems.

First, the resection or cutting away of prostate tissue may not have been sufficient to relieve the urinary symptoms. Occasionally it will be necessary to cut away further tissue, usually by repeating the TURP procedure. Sometimes relief is adequate for a few months or years, but further enlargement of the prostate might mean the patient will need a further resection by TURP.

The second problem is not a consequence of the operation itself. It may be that the pathologist finds cancer cells in some of the prostate tissue removed. In this situation further treatment will depend on many circumstances. Sometimes, if relief of symptoms has been achieved, especially if the patient is elderly and otherwise not well, it may be best to wait and see whether further treatment is needed.

The third problem that occasionally arises after the TURP operation is incomplete control of bladder emptying and urinary incontinence or dribbling. An exercise program to strengthen pelvic muscle tissue can help to improve control, but the problem can persist for several weeks or longer. Until this has settled it can be advisable for the man to wear a pad in his underpants. Pads specially made to help people live with this problem are com-monly used by men and women with stress incontinence or occasional incontinence quite unrelated to any surgical procedure. The pads are inexpensive and are readily available in chemist shops. A small adhesive tape keeps them securely in position.

Some men will find that they have sexual difficulties after a TURP operation that they did not have before the operation. These difficulties might include loss of interest in sex or the inability to obtain an erection in spite of a desire. These men and their partners need to be reassured that these problems are usually temporary. Provided they are prepared to wait and don't become overanxious, there is no physical reason why the TURP operation should have changed their sex life. If the problem continues, then the help of a sex counsellor could be advisable. Occasionally standard methods of treatment for sex problems after radical prostatectomy (as discussed in chapter 14) could be the most helpful solution.

Non-surgical treatment

Until recently, surgery was the only realistic treatment option for benign hyperplasia of the prostate that was causing problems with passage of urine. The only other option was the largely unacceptable practice of passing a catheter either repeatedly or for a long period.

In recent years an effective muscle-relaxing medication called prazosin (brand name Minipress) has become available. Prazosin relaxes the muscle in the prostate and relaxes the tight muscle around the exit passage from the bladder (the bladder neck) and so allows urine to pass more freely from the bladder and through the urethra passing through the prostate. A newer agent called terazosin (brand name Hytrin) may be more effective in some cases.

Another new drug, finasteride (brand name Proscar), can often help in a different way. Finasteride blocks the conversion in the body of the male hormone testosterone into dihydrotestosterone, the more active form of the hormone. Testosterone can stimulate the prostate, causing it to enlarge, but in its more active form of dihydrotestosterone this stimulation is much stronger. By blocking the conversion of testosterone to dihydrotestosterone, finasteride reduces the stimulus to prostate enlargement and often results in some shrinkage or reduction in size of the prostate. This reduction in size can be up to 20 per cent.

With very large prostates the size reduction achieved by taking finasteride may be enough to give good relief of symptoms related to blockage of the flow of urine. The main problem is that a man who does get good relief with this medication must continue to take finasteride tablets for the rest of his life; otherwise symptoms are likely to recur. The other problem is that with the reduction of male hormones there may be a reduction in sex drive or even impotence, although impotence can now be treated in other ways, as will be described later in this book.

Which treatment should be used?

For a man with troublesome urinary symptoms which have been shown to be caused by benign hyperplasia of the prostate, a decision must be made as to whether the man's symptoms justify treatment, considering his age and general state of health. If the symptoms do require treatment, the best choice of treatment needs to be decided.

The first choice that must be made is between surgical (that is, operative) treatment (usually the TURP operation) or conservative (that is, non-operative) treatment. Until recently there was no choice, but now that medications that may be effective are available and they can be given simply in tablet form, the first choice of treatment may be to use medications, at least for a trial period.

The placebo effect

The results of studies in which drugs are used to treat medical conditions are often somewhat exaggerated by what is called the placebo effect. It is well recognised that some patients will report feeling better after they have been given treatment, even if the treatment given was known to have no medical value; that is, it was a placebo, an inactive agent used to compare with an active drug under investigation.

In studies of the effectiveness of a new drug, it is usual practice to explain to the patients in the trial that they may not be given the active drug that is being tested. Half the people in the trial will be given the drug being tested, and half will be given an inactive agent (placebo) that looks the same. The patients are not told which they are given. A proportion of the people given the placebo will still report an improvement. This is called the 'placebo effect' and may be experienced by as many as 25 per cent of patients in that group. The apparent benefit is due to psychological and emotional factors and a great wish to be able to report a benefit, but usually the placebo effect does not last long. The benefit will not be great and will not continue for weeks or months.

In using drugs or medication to treat men for symptoms of hyperplasia, the possibility of an apparent benefit merely from having treatment, the 'placebo effect', must be kept in mind, no matter what drug the patient is given. This is why giving medication for a trial period, with follow-up assessment, is important: in such a case any apparent benefit may not be long-lasting.

Which medications to use?

Depending on the size of the prostate when it is felt by digital examination, the doctor will usually advise whether to try a muscle-relaxing agent (like prazosin or terazosin) first or whether to try an agent to shrink the prostate (like finasteride).

If the prostate is not very big or is only moderately enlarged, it might suggest that tightness of the muscle tissue in the prostate or in the neck of the bladder is largely responsible for the symptoms. The most suitable agent to try first would then seem to be a muscle-relaxing agent like prazosin or terazosin.

If the prostate is found to be very big it is more likely that its size is largely responsible for the obstruction to flow of urine. It would then seem that an agent to reduce the size of the prostate would be best to try first. Finasteride would then be tried first.

In both cases, if the agent first tried does not give satisfactory relief of symptoms, then the other type of agent is tried.

If benign prostate hyperplasia is causing troublesome urinary difficulty and symptoms are not sufficiently relieved by any medications, then surgery is likely to be recommended, usually a TURP operation.

Case report 1: *Bill, aged 59*

Bill was a farmer aged 59 who had never had a day's serious illness prior to having a heart attack and coronary artery bypass surgery three years earlier. He now came to his doctor complaining of increasing difficulty in passing urine and frequency that required him to get out of bed three or four times at night to pass urine. The doctor's examination included a digital examination of the rectum, at which he found a large smooth prostate gland. The doctor arranged for a specimen of blood to be taken on another day for a full blood count (which might show up or eliminate other possible health problems) and also a PSA test.

The PSA test was reported as 6.1, which is slightly raised for Bill's age, so the doctor arranged for Bill to see a specialist urologist.

The urologist repeated the examinations and confirmed the family doctor's findings. The urologist therefore arranged for an ultrasound study of Bill's prostate. The ultrasound did not show any lump in the prostate gland, but during the ultrasound examination three biopsies were taken from each side of the prostate. No cancer was found. The urologist explained to Bill that he had benign hyperplasia (that is, a simple enlargement of the prostate gland), but there was no evidence of cancer. The urologist then recommended a trial treatment by medication, without an operation.

The family doctor prescribed the prostate-shrinking drug Proscar. This gave Bill considerable improvement in symptoms for a year, but then the same symptoms of urine obstruction returned. The doctor then recommended a trial of the muscle-relaxing drug Minipress. Again symptoms were improved for several months, but then they recurred.

By this time Bill's PSA had increased to 7.2, so the digital examination and ultrasound tests were repeated. Again no cancer was detected. The urologist then recommended TURP (resection or cutting away the part of the prostate causing the obstruction). Microscopic examination by a skilled pathologist of the tissue removed showed no evidence of cancer and three years later Bill remains well, free of symptoms and sexually active, but he is kept under regular observation with a PSA check and digital examination every six or twelve months.

7

General aspects of prostate cancer

Cancer of the prostate is uncommon before the age of 50 but it is the most common internal cancer in men over the age of 65. It became increasingly common in Western societies during the twentieth century.

The cause of prostate cancer is unknown, but its association with old age is illustrated by the fact that almost all men over the age of 90 have microscopic evidence of at least early prostate cancer.

Prostate cancer is less common in some Asian, African, South American and Mediterranean countries than it is in most Western countries. As discussed in chapter 4, it is likely that differences in diet may be significant, as prostate cancer is less common in communities that have predominantly vegetarian diets than it is in communities that have diets high in animal products. Diets with a high content of legumes, such as soya beans, and diets with a high content of tomatoes, especially tomato pastes or cooked tomatoes, may be protective. It seems that lycopene (the natural red colouring matter in tomatoes) and the high content in soya and other legumes of naturally occurring plant hormones (the phytoestrogens and especially the isoflavones) and related compounds could be responsible.

Presentation

Nowadays prostate cancer is commonly detected before it has caused any symptoms. The first indication of cancer may be the finding of a raised PSA index when the PSA is done as a routine screening test, but sometimes the first indication is the doctor finding a hard or lumpy prostate gland when a digital rectal examination is done for other reasons.

As discussed previously, the most common clinical presentation of prostate cancer—the symptom that drives most men to see their doctor—is difficulty passing urine. Any man with a history of urinary symptoms should see his family doctor. In general men will not mention symptoms of any potentially serious problem as readily as women do. Most men are especially reluctant to mention or discuss any symptoms that might appear to question their self-image of their 'manhood' or 'virility', and the most obvious of these self-image symptoms are symptoms possibly associated with the sexual organs.

If a man presents himself to his doctor with a history of frequency, difficulty, dribbling, or other urinary symptoms, the doctor will ask more questions about his ability to pass urine and will want to carry out a digital examination of the rectum to feel the prostate. The doctor will particularly observe the size, shape and consistency (softness or hardness), and any nodularity or lumpiness or tenderness of the prostate. At the same time the doctor will note the normality or abnormality of any other contents of the pelvis or in the rectum that can be felt with the examining finger.

Non-malignant enlargement of the prostate (benign prostatic hyperplasia) is more often the cause of urinary difficulty than is cancer, but prostate cancer is also a common cause, especially in older men. Urinary infection and frequency is also sometimes a feature of prostate cancer. The frequency is due to the cancer obstructing the flow of urine and thus failing to allow complete emptying of the bladder.

Occasionally the first evidence of prostate cancer is due to secondary tumours (metastases), most often appearing in bone and causing bone pain or fractures. Secondaries in the lower vertebral column (backbone) or pelvis may cause pressure on the main nerve to the leg, the sciatic nerve, causing severe pain in the back and leg, called sciatica. Sciatica is more often caused by other conditions, but occasionally it is the first evidence of a prostate cancer.

Investigations and special tests

If the symptoms described above are present or if a PSA test result is significantly raised, it is advisable to have further examination and investigations.

Digital rectal examination (DRE)

The prostate gland can be felt by the examining finger when a doctor does a DRE (digital rectal examination). That is, a gloved finger is passed through the anus into the rectum and the prostate gland can be felt in front of the finger (see figure 2.1). Cancer in the prostate feels like a hard lump in the prostate, or sometimes the whole of the prostate gland may feel hard and rigid instead of having its normal rubbery texture.

Biopsy of the prostate gland

Sometimes small biopsies of prostate tissue can be taken with a needle passed through the skin in front of the anus and guided by a finger in the rectum, but nowadays the biopsies are usually taken through the anus with a needle or punch instrument passed through a small hollow tube that the doctor inserts through a wider tube in the anus (an anal speculum). The needle or punch is pushed through the wall of the lower rectum into the back of the prostate gland. The biopsies are usually taken with a spring-loaded punch instrument that causes the patient to hear a bang and to feel a sudden jolt, rather like an electric shock, but the procedure is usually not painful. Usually about six biopsy specimens are taken within a minute or two and these are sent to a pathologist for special microscopic examination. The pathologist's examination and report is usually completed in four or five days.

In most clinics ultrasound is used to help guide the biopsy needle or punch into the parts of the prostate under suspicion of harbouring a possible malignancy. The ultrasound instrument has a special small probe that is passed through the anus into the rectum. Ultrasound will show any lumps in the prostate and any general prostate enlargement, so it helps indicate the places in the prostate where any cancer is most likely to be present and therefore the places from which it is best to take the biopsies. When biopsies are taken through the wall of the rectum it is advisable that the rectum should have been emptied before the test. A liquid diet for 24 hours followed by a suppository a few hours before the test will usually suffice. It is also important for the procedure to be made as clean as possible by the patient taking some antibiotics by mouth before and after the biopsy procedure.

Biopsy may sometimes also be required to determine whether a mass in bone, lung, liver, lymph node or other tissue is a prostate cancer secondary (metastasis). Often such biopsies can be carried out without needing a major procedure or a general anaesthetic; this will depend on the site and nature of the biopsy being performed.

X-rays

X-rays will be taken to look for evidence of secondary (metastatic) spread into bones. If secondary cancers are present they may show as areas of bone loss or bone destruction but they more commonly show up as dense white (sclerotic) areas in the bone because they usually contain more calcium than normal bone. Chest X-rays may show evidence of secondaries in the lungs, in lymph nodes in the chest, or even in the ribs. Isotope bone scans are also valuable in showing evidence of bone secondaries. The isotope scans (something like special X-rays) require a small amount of the isotope material to be injected into a vein before the procedure.

Bone scans

A bone scan is something like an X-ray. A radioactive substance is injected into the bloodstream and goes into the bones. The radioactivity in the bones is then recorded outside the body on film or on a television screen.

In this procedure, two or three hours before the scans can be taken the patient is given a very small injection of a radioactive substance called technetium. The injection is given into a vein in the arm. The technetium in the circulation takes about two or three hours to reach its maximum concentration in the bones. Recordings are then taken by a type of camera positioned over the patient, who simply lies on a recording couch. The technician records pictures of the whole bony skeleton and then asks the patient to lie in different positions so that magnified images can be taken from different angles and of bones of special concern.

Excessive radioactivity detected in any part of bone is an indication of increased activity of cells and tissues at that site. In a man with prostate cancer, excessive activity (called a 'hot spot') is likely to be a deposit of growing cancer cells (a metastasis or secondary) (see figure 7.1).

Apart from the initial pinprick for the injection of radioactive technetium, the whole bone scan procedure is painless. After the wait for the technetium to reach the bones, the scanning takes less than an hour, and results of the test should be ready in a day or two.

It is important for bone scan testing to be carried out before any major prostate surgery is planned in an attempt at cure. The presence of secondaries in bones makes it impossible to cure the cancer by surgery. However, if the prostate is causing obstruction to the flow of urine a TURP (trans-urethral resection of the prostate) of the tissue causing the blockage will often relieve the patient of his most immediate distressing symptoms.

Bones containing 'hot spots' may be X-rayed to reveal more evidence and information about the bone damage. Prostate secondaries in bones usually are seen in X-rays as sclerotic or 'white areas' of damage due to the calcium usually present in those bone secondaries (see figure 2.3 and figure 7.1). For prostate secondaries in bones, some form of hormone treatment is probably appropriate. Any cancer that has recurred in the prostate region after surgical removal of the prostate may also be treated by radiation therapy, but this is not an option if radiation therapy was originally used to treat the cancer in the prostate. A second dose of radiation treatment should not be given to the same area of body tissue because it would cause excessive tissue damage.

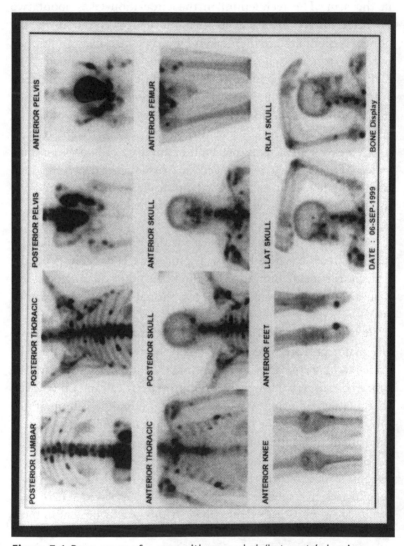

Figure 7.1 Bone scans of a man with many dark 'hot spots' showing prostate cancer secondaries in bones. The big dark area in the pelvis is due to the radioactive technetium excreted by the kidneys and held in the urine in the bladder until the bladder is next emptied.

Blood studies

Blood tests may show evidence of anaemia due to bone secondaries destroying the blood-forming cells in bone marrow. Cancer of the prostate may also cause an elevation of an enzyme in blood called acid phosphatase, and if bone is destroyed by secondary tumours, an enzyme released from the bone called alkaline phosphatase may also be elevated. These tests and the PSA test are all made on a small specimen of a few millilitres of blood taken from a vein before the prostate has been pressed by the doctor's examining finger.

Obstruction by the cancer to the flow of urine may cause infection in the bladder and possibly in the kidneys. The urine and blood are examined for evidence of infection and for evidence of damage to the kidneys. If infection is found it will be treated accordingly.

Not all of these investigations are necessarily done in every patient, as needs and presentation will be different in different patients. For example, if a man presents with acute obstruction of urine and pain, emergency procedures to relieve the obstruction will be required before biopsies to establish its cause have been taken.

What treatments are available?

There are at present only two known methods of treating prostate cancer that offer any chance of totally eradicating the cancer to achieve a cure. One is surgery, and the other is radiation therapy (radiotherapy). Whether either of these, or any other active treatment, is advisable is a matter requiring special consideration for each patient.

A third option is 'watchful waiting'. This simply means that the doctor keeps the patient under regular observation before deciding whether any attempt at cure—or indeed any treatment at all—is necessary. This strategy can be hard for patients and their families to understand, as we are used to being told that early detection and treatment of cancer is essential for cure. However, with prostate cancer it may be that the patient has one of those 'latent cancers' that can lie dormant or progress only very slowly without much bothering the patient before a more rapid health problem or old age takes his life. If surgery in the prostate area were as simple as removing a suspicious-looking skin blemish, with no serious after-effects, then doctors would be more willing to operate. However, as described in chapter 8, surgery to remove the prostate is difficult, and the operation can have serious effects on the quality of the patient's future life. Radiotherapy is not a simple treatment either, and it too can have lasting effects on the patient's quality of life.

Men being cared for with 'watchful waiting' are advised to return for a PSA and a digital examination of the prostate every six months or so, or sooner if there is any significant change in symptoms. It should be noted that if a PSA and digital examination are to be performed at the one visit or on the same day, the blood is probably better taken for the PSA before the digital examination is performed. This is in case the PSA is raised to an artificially high level as a result of the doctor pressing on the prostate gland. Although there is doubt about whether this happens and so whether the precaution is really necessary, it is the reason why doctors prefer to take the resting blood measurement of PSA on blood taken before the digital examination and not immediately after, when it may be artificially raised.

8

Surgical treatment

An operation can be used in treatment of prostate cancer with one or more of the following objectives:
• to establish a diagnosis
• to relieve symptoms of pain or discomfort or obstruction of urinary flow
• to remove the cancer totally and achieve a cure.

Surgery to establish a diagnosis

Before carrying out major surgery on the prostate with a view to curing the cancer, it is important for the surgeon to know as accurately as possible whether the cancer has spread, including whether lymph nodes near the prostate are involved with secondary cancer. The surgeon therefore takes biopsies of nearby lymph nodes and has them examined before proceeding with the complete removal of the prostate gland, a major operation called radical prostatectomy.

It takes two to three days to get the pathology results from a routine biopsy. For a routine examination, the specimen is set in a solid wax block, which takes some time to set hard enough to be sliced thinly for staining and examination under a microscope. However, if the extent of surgery depends on the presence or absence of cancer cells in lymph nodes, for example, it is important for the surgeon to know immediately whether cancer cells are present in the tissue. A technique called a *frozen section*, in which the biopsy specimen is immediately frozen solid, cut and stained for microscopic examination, allows the pathologist to give the surgeon results in a few minutes.

If the pathologist or surgeon discovers that the cancer has spread to lymph nodes some distance from the prostate, it is unlikely that the cancer will be totally removable. It therefore cannot be cured by surgery. In this case a decision will probably be made not to proceed further with the operation but to use another method of treatment instead.

Surgery to relieve symptoms

The most common operation in treating prostate cancer is to relieve obstruction to the flow of urine. The surgery is intended to relieve symptoms of difficulty or pain on passing urine, urinary incontinence, urinary frequency or sometimes complete urinary obstruction.

Usually prostate surgery of this type is performed with the patient under a general anaesthetic but a spinal anaesthetic is sometimes preferred. A long, slim, flexible instrument called a resectoscope is passed up the urethra, the passage in the penis. The surgeon can see the the site of obstruction through a series of mirrors and lenses and is able to cut it away with this diathermy cutting instrument. This procedure, called a TURP (trans–urethral resection of prostate), is more commonly used to relieve these symptoms in men with urinary obstruction caused by prostatic hyperplasia, which is a more common cause of cause of urinary obstruction than cancer. The procedure has been described in detail in chapter 6, in the discussion of hyperplasia. Nonetheless, whenever tissue is removed with a resectoscope, even for benign disease, it is always sent to a pathologist for microscopic examination in case cancer cells are present.

Patients should be advised that some bleeding always occurs after a TURP resection. This is normal for a few days but soon settles. Patients should also be advised that sometimes a further TURP resection may be required at a later date if their urinary difficulties recur. They are also advised not to take aspirin for at least ten days before and for two or three weeks after any cutting procedure is to be carried out, as aspirin increases the risk of excessive bleeding.

Surgery for cure

There is as yet no way of determining for sure whether operation for prostate cancer, or indeed any treatment, is essential, as not all prostate cancers will progress during the patient's likely period of life expectancy. This is the most difficult point for consideration.

If a prostate cancer has been diagnosed in its early stages and before it has spread beyond the confines of the prostate gland, and the patient is young enough and fit enough to undergo major surgery, consideration should be given to carrying out total (radical) surgical removal of the prostate with the objective, and every probability, of achieving a cure. However, this procedure should not be undertaken lightly, as it is a major and difficult surgical operation. It requires a highly skilled surgeon and surgical team and competent post-operative nursing care. The patient must be willing to accept post-operative incontinence of urine possibly for some weeks or months, and other likely complications, including sexual impotence.

Radical prostatectomy

Preparing for surgery

Although blood transfusions are still required during radical prostatectomy, improvements in surgical techniques mean that the quantity needed is normally fairly small, equivalent to three blood donations (three units). With modern extra-safe blood transfusions it is common practice for the man's own blood to be used. Arrangements can usually be made with the hospital's blood transfusion service for the patient to visit the hospital for an hour or so on three separate occasions at two-week intervals, finishing one or two weeks before the planned operation. At each visit a unit of his own blood is taken and kept in storage for use during and after the operation. Alternatively, the patient's doctor may arrange for the patient's own blood to be collected by the Red Cross at a blood bank.

Using the patient's own blood in this way avoids any possible risks associated with being transfused with someone else's blood.

After hospital admission

The patient will usually be admitted to hospital one or two days before the planned date of the operation.

In hospital, a lot of attention will be given to cleaning out the bowel and to leaving any remaining contents as sterile as possible. An empty bowel gives more room for the surgeon to operate, and a sterile bowel is a safety precaution in case of injury to the rectum during the operation. The cleaning of the bowel is not pleasant. The patient is given a large amount of clear fluid to drink, probably containing glycerine or a mixture of 'salts'. After that he feels the need to pay frequent and urgent visits to the toilet to empty his bowels. He is given no solid food, but only clear broth, fruit juices, jellies, and perhaps some ice-cream. He is, however, allowed as much water, tea and coffee as he wants.

A course of antibiotics is started to help make the operation and post-operative procedures as clean and sterile as possible, to avoid any risk of infection.

Nursing staff will be familiar with all these requirements and can help allay the patient's anxieties. A visit from the surgeon and anaesthetist will allow any further questions to be answered.

Usually a sleeping tablet is given in the evening before the surgery and usually a calming or tranquillising tablet will be prescribed, even if it is not requested by the patient. Nothing further should be taken by mouth by the patient for 8 to 12 hours prior to surgery. An hour or so before operation with a standard anaesthetic, a 'premedication'—a tranquillising or calming injection—is also given.

Difficulties with the operation

The complex operation to remove a prostate gland is difficult to carry out because the prostate is very difficult to reach. The pubic bone is right in front of it, the bladder is right on top of it, and the rectum is right behind it. In other words, the prostate is 'jammed into' this tight little space (see figure 2.1). As well as this, the prostate is surrounded by a rich network of fragile blood vessels that bleed profusely when injured.

To add to the difficulties for the surgical team, the urethra, the important passage for urine to pass from the bladder to the penis, runs through the middle of the prostate. When the prostate is removed, so is a section of about two or three centimetres of the urethra. The two ends of the cut urethra must then be rejoined to allow urine to pass through again—with the same difficulties of a tight space to work in and lots of small blood vessels ready to bleed. If bleeding is not well controlled it all becomes too difficult to see.

In the past a great deal of blood loss was inevitable with this operation, and this is one reason it was rarely performed. Several litres of blood were required for transfusion during and after the operation. Fortunately new techniques are used to control the likely blood flow by temporarily clamping or temporarily tying off important blood vessels early in the operation, before the actual removal of the prostate has started. These techniques allow the operation to be performed with much more safety, and so in recent years it has become more common.

The reason for explaining the operation in some detail in this book is so that the reader will understand why radical prostatectomy was rarely accepted as a reasonable risk by most of the medical profession until the newer and safer techniques were developed. Even now it is most important that a surgeon with special skills and experience in this type of surgery be selected to do this operation. It is not a job for every surgeon to do from time to time, but a demanding task that requires a highly experienced surgeon who is prepared to specialise in this area.

Immediately after the operation

The patient will wake after operation in a special 'recovery' or intensive-care ward in the hospital. Here he will wake finding that he is surrounded by special monitoring equipment recording his pulse, blood pressure, heart function (electrocardiogram), and other important measurements. There will be drips of fluid or possibly blood going into one or two veins, possibly another monitoring tube in an artery, a drainage tube in his abdominal wound, and a catheter in his penis. Very likely there will also be a fine tube in his back delivering a slow drip of a pain-relieving agent (an 'epidural', often given to women to relieve the pain of delivering a baby). Only his wife or other close members of his family are allowed to visit him in the intensive-care ward, but after a day or two he is moved back into his regular hospital ward where a full range of friends may visit.

One by one the various monitoring and other tubes are removed. Initially the only things he is allowed to swallow are fluids, but these are gradually increased and the range expanded to allow soft foods. If all goes well a good diet is restored after a few days, when there has been passage of wind or other evidence that the bowels are ready to work again.

Post-operative problems

Short-term care

When the patient is able to go home a week or so after surgery, he will be up and about and quite mobile. He should be back to his normal diet with normal bowel movements, and will be free of all tubes except for the tube through his penis and into his bladder. This may stay for possibly three weeks or so to support the urethra until it is well healed. The patient will learn to keep a special plastic bag strapped to his thigh or leg, out of sight, and urine from the catheter dribbles into it. The plastic bag needs to be emptied when it fills, perhaps two or three times a day.

After about three weeks or so it should be time for the catheter in the bladder to be removed. An appointment is made for X-rays to be taken in an X-ray department experienced in this work. The patient lies on a specially equipped X-ray table while an amount of a special fluid (often called 'dye') is slowly injected up the catheter and into the bladder. After possibly 150 to 300 millilitres of the dye has been injected the patient will say that his bladder feels full, and then the X-rays will be taken. This 'radio-opaque' fluid shows up strongly on the X-rays and so maps out the shape of the bladder and the urethra. The X-rays will show whether the bladder appears to have returned to its normal size and shape, but especially whether the repair of the urethra appears to have been successful and is apparently complete. If the X-rays show the repair is complete the patient should be ready to have the indwelling catheter removed. If healing is not complete then the catheter is left for a longer period.

If the surgeon is satisfied that healing of the urethra is satisfactory the catheter will be removed, usually by an experienced nurse.

At first the patient will have lost control of his bladder, and urine will dribble into a tube or a pad that he must wear. However, things do get better. The patient will be taught pelvic muscle strengthening exercises that he should practise until control of his bladder function and emptying of urine returns—possibly in a month or so. Control should improve further as time passes but an occasional little dribble is almost inevitable, especially when the man is tired or at times of mental or physical stress. It is usually advisable for him to wear or carry a pad ready to insert into his underpants if these occasions arise.

If urine does not flow well after prostatectomy or if there is a lot of pain passing urine (this has been graphically described as 'like pissing razor blades'), it may be due to narrowing or stricture of the urethra at the site of its repair. This trouble can usually be fixed fairly simply by the surgeon passing a dilating instrument, called a 'sound', through the narrow stricture to stretch it. This is a simple and safe procedure, but a short general anaesthetic will be required.

Long-term problems

After radical prostatectomy the man will be sterile.

The most distressing and consistent post-operative complication is sexual impotence. However, there are ways of overcoming sexual impotence in most patients. These are described in chapter 14.

Of course, as for any cancer, cure cannot be guaranteed, but the prospects of cure by a properly considered and skilfully carried out prostatectomy are very good.

After prostatectomy, if the operation has been successful in curing the cancer, the patient's PSA should fall to almost zero and remain very low thereafter. An elevated PSA indicates that some cancer tissue remains. It is bad news if after prostatectomy the PSA falls to almost zero but later starts to rise again. It suggests almost certain recurrence of the cancer.

Case report 2: *Frank, aged 67*

Frank was a retired soldier, very fit and active for his age. He had no urinary symptoms but his doctor had included a PSA in a routine health check and this was found to be 6.5. Frank was referred to a specialist urologist. The urologist found Frank's prostate to be moderately enlarged but no lumps were felt. He was advised to have a further check in six months.

On his next visit Frank was still free of symptoms but his PSA was 7.2. The urologist's findings were unchanged—there were still no lumps that could be felt—but an ultrasound was arranged and six biopsies were taken, three from each side of Frank's prostate.

The biopsy report described low-grade 'latent' cancer cells in one of the six biopsy specimens. The specialist explained that treatment would certainly risk impotence and other side effects, and so recommended follow-up examinations at six-month intervals.

Frank decided that he did not want any active treatment. He has been regularly followed up for six years and remains well. Now he is aged 73, his PSA has gradually risen to 8.8 and his prostate has become a little larger, but apart from getting out of bed to pass urine once or twice at night Frank has no urological symptoms. Frank and his wife still enjoy an active sex life.

Case report 3: *George, aged 65*

George was a teacher who had a regular annual health check by his family doctor. At his latest check a raised PSA of 6.2 was found. George was otherwise well and did not complain of any urinary symptoms.

His doctor arranged a consultation with a specialist urologist who felt a prostate that was firm but not particularly enlarged, and no lumps were felt. An ultrasound test did not show any lump, but three biopsies were taken from either side of the prostate gland. The biopsies were all negative for cancer.

One year later the tests were all repeated. The PSA had risen to 8.1, and the ultrasound showed a small nodular area in the left lobe of the prostate gland. Biopsy of this area showed a small collection of low-grade malignant cells in one specimen from the left lobe of the prostate gland.

It was explained to George that the few positive cells might represent low-grade 'latent' cancer that might not progress, and that any form of treatment would risk complications and in particular would be likely to make him impotent. After discussion between George, his doctor and the urologist, it was decided to repeat all tests in four months.

In four months the PSA had risen to 9.2. Biopsies showed positive cancer cells in two specimens with slightly higher-grade cells in one specimen.

George was otherwise fit and well with an otherwise good life expectancy. In view of the apparent progress of the malignant cells, which still seemed to be contained in the prostate gland only and therefore appeared curable, George and his wife decided on radical prostatectomy as his preferred choice of treatment.

The operation was performed without any major problem other than a rather prolonged period before George had complete control of his urine. However, since the operation George failed to achieve a satisfactory erection in spite of his urge to have intercourse.

After discussion between the urologist and the family doctor, George was shown how to inject his penis with prostaglandins, and using these he achieved satisfactory intercourse without ejaculation but with good orgasm.

As injection of the penis is rather painful and unpleasant, George has used both Viagra and Muse to try to achieve an erection. With both he achieved an erection on most but not all occasions, but the penile injections were more reliable and very much less expensive.

George has remained well for all six years since his operation. He and his wife are having a satisfactory sex life. George's PSA has been virtually zero since the operation and there is almost a guarantee that his prostate cancer has been cured.

9

Radiotherapy

Like surgery, radiotherapy (radiation therapy) can be used in treatment of prostate cancer with the objective of cure. Radiotherapy may also be used with the objective of good palliation or relief of distressing symptoms.

The radiation kills cells by damaging the DNA in the cell nucleus. All cells can be damaged by radiation, which is why the treatment has to be controlled very precisely, but the type of cancer cells found in prostate cancer are more easily killed by radiation than are healthy cells.

Radiotherapy for cure

Two techniques of radiotherapy can be used in treating prostate cancer. The most common, and standard, treatment is with the use of modern external deep penetrating irradiation. Present techniques use linear accelerator high-energy irradiation equipment that is available only at hospitals or institutions with specialised radiation oncology units. Computer models assist in planning the best irradiation 'fields'; that is, the size, areas to be covered, direction of irradiation beams, doses to be given etc.

Simulation

When the patient first attends a radiation therapy department (if it specialises in cancer treatment it may be called a radiation oncology department) he will be taken to a 'simulator room' for what is called the simulation. There he will be introduced to technical staff who will take X-rays of the parts of the body to be treated. They will plan with great precision and accuracy how much irradiation should be given from different angles to achieve the maximum effect on the part containing the cancer while at the same time causing the minimum damage to surrounding and overlying normal tissues and cells. Little tattoo marks will be made in the skin so that for each treatment given on the following days the radiotherapy technician will know exactly where to direct the irradiation. These pinhead-sized tattoo marks remain, and are there to avoid the need to repeat the calculation of plans for treatment on each treatment visit.

The whole process of simulation is done only on the first visit and should take no more than one hour. The tiny tattoo marks avoid the need to repeat it. Like any other tattoos, these small spots remain in the skin permanently, but because they are so small they are not conspicuous and in fact are not always easy to find.

Delivery of radiotherapy

In most radiotherapy departments the treatment is given only four or five days in each week. Weekends are free, and one day every second week is set aside for servicing the intricate equipment.

In the treatment room the patient will be asked to lie on the treatment couch. Using the tattoo marks as a guide, the technician will help the patient to get into the best position so that treatment will be delivered in exactly the right direction. The patient is made comfortable and is asked to keep still but to breathe normally.

The radiographer will then go into an adjoining room. This has a glass window so that a close watch can be kept on the patient. An installed microphone system allows the patient and the radiographer to continue to talk to each other. The reason the technician giving treatment must stay out of the treatment room while irradiation is being delivered is that, although the dose of irradiation scattered around the room is very small, the technician is doing this work almost every day for his or her working life. Over this period the accumulation of even small doses of irradiation would become dangerous.

When the treatment equipment is switched on, the patient will hear a soft whining noise. The active head of the machine will move around the patient's body, delivering exactly the right amount of irradiation over the right period of time in the right directions to the right parts of the body, or 'fields', as previously calculated. It is a remarkably precise process designed to give the maximum benefit by destroying cancer cells with the minimum of damage to other tissues. The whole treatment process will take less than half an hour on each treatment day, and the actual delivery of irradiation is only for a part of that time. The treatment takes seven or eight weeks to complete.

The precision equipment and computerised designs ensure that the maximum safe and effective doses are given to the cancer region with as little damage as possible to the rectum, bladder and other nearby tissues. The objective is for the cancer cells to be repeatedly bombarded with a dose of irradiation from which they cannot recover, but to keep any damage to normal tissues or cells small and to an extent from which they can readily recover.

Some radiotherapy studies have indicated that the cure rate from radiotherapy can nearly match the cure rate from surgery for cancers localised in the prostate gland. An advantage of radiotherapy is that it is much easier for the patient to tolerate than a major surgical operation. It also has the advantage that it gives very good localised palliative treatment and possibly a cure for patients in whom the cancer has spread beyond the confines of the prostate and its surrounding membranes and so is not able to be removed completely by surgery.

Side effects

Some people become fatigued and others become psychologically and emotionally depressed during the course of radiation therapy. They should recover from these effects in two or three weeks or possibly a little longer after radiotherapy has been completed.

The skin over the field of irradiation will sometimes become dry, reddish, itchy, and sensitive. Sunbaking or dry heat such as provided by electric blankets will make it worse and should be avoided. Soaps or drying agents like alcohol wipes, aftershaves or perfumes should also be avoided on irradiated skin. Baths or showers should be tepid or just warm enough to be comfortable, but not hot. A moisturising lotion is often helpful. The patient should avoid tight or woollen clothing and preferably should wear loose cotton clothing.

As with surgery, impotence is almost inevitable after full-dose radiotherapy. If lack of sexual desire persists or impotence does develop and is present for some months, it is likely to be permanent. However, there are now several possible treatments for both lack of sexual desire and impotence, as discussed in chapter 14. The patient may wish to try one or more of these treatments but should only do so under the guidance of his doctor or other expert. He may wish to get advice from a sex therapist provided his doctor or specialist radiotherapist thinks it would be appropriate.

The other chief worry is that the rectum and bladder cannot be completely protected from irradiation, and some patients are left with some degree of precipitous diarrhoea, sometimes with bleeding, or even bowel incontinence. Urinary discomfort, frequency, burning, and loss of good control can also result, but these symptoms, which often start after two or three irradiation treatments, usually settle in a month or two after irradiation therapy has been completed.

The problems of diarrhoea may need temporary or long-term adjustment to diet (less bran, less fruit and vegetable, less fibre and roughage). Some medication may be needed for several weeks, but the doctor will need to give advice to patients on an individual basis as symptoms will be different in different patients.

Brachytherapy

The other technique of radiation therapy is called brachytherapy. This is a method of directing radiation right into the cancer itself by inserting wires or seeds (tiny pellets) containing radioactive materials directly into the prostate gland.

These techniques are still being developed and not all problems have yet been solved, but experts experienced in these techniques are usually enthusiastic about their use and future potential. One considerable potential advantage of brachytherapy is that the irradiation is directed precisely to the prostate gland and cancer tissue. This means it can be given in greater concentration than can external irradiation, without the same risk of damaging the rectum or bladder or other nearby tissues. A disadvantage is that without extremely accurate planting of the irradiation materials some cancer cells may escape the irradiation. Nor will the irradiation field cover those lymph nodes and other nearby tissues that might contain some malignant cells.

There are two main methods of administering brachytherapy. One is by implanting seeds containing a preparation of radioiodine directly into the cancer region of the prostate gland. These seeds remain in place permanently and emit a measured dose of irradiation directly into the cancer region for as long as they remain radioactive. They thus must be placed accurately into exactly the right position and the dose of irradiation must be calculated with great accuracy. There is little penetration of the nearby organs like bladder and rectum by the irradiation, so these organs receive very little irradiation and suffer little damage. Impotence is unlikely to be a problem but there may be some temporary damage to the urethra where it passes through the prostate, resulting in temporary discomfort and frequency in passing urine. Due to the very localised activity with little penetration of these implanted seeds this treatment is not suitable for locally advanced cancers. It is also a very expensive form of treatment.

The other form of brachytherapy is with radioactive wires implanted into and through the prostate gland and cancer. These wires are left in place until the required measured dose of irradiation has been completed. The wires are then removed. The position of these wires can be adjusted if necessary. This form of treatment concentrates radiation to the cancer region but penetration to surrounding lymph nodes or other tissues possibly involved in the cancer is limited.

Combined external radiotherapy and brachytherapy

Some centres treating locally advanced cancers combine brachytherapy with conventional externally delivered radiotherapy.
Studies suggest that especially for locally advanced cancers this
treatment may be more effective than radical surgery, and for less
advanced cancers the results are believed to be comparable to those
achieved by surgery. Standard external irradiation at a measured
but slightly reduced dose is often given first and this is followed by
brachytherapy with implanted radioactive wires directly into the
cancer site. Although irradiation damage to the bladder or rectum
can still be a problem, impotence is less likely than with full-dose
standard external irradiation. Experts in these techniques believe
their results can now match the results achieved by radical surgery
with fewer troublesome side effects.

Follow up

It is important for the doctors to arrange regular follow-up
consultations after any form of radiation therapy, especially to
determine how effective the radiotherapy has been in curing the
cancer.

The two main follow-up tests are regular digital rectal examinations for any evidence of recurrence of cancer in the
prostate, and regular PSA tests for evidence of regrowth of prostate
cancer cells. If either of these is positive then bone scans or bone
X-rays or other tests for the presence of metastases may be
performed.

Further treatment possibilities if the cancer has reappeared may
include irradiation to one or two sites of secondaries in bone, or a
more general treatment such as one of the forms of hormone
treatment. Further radiation treatment cannot be given to the
prostate region as the maximum safe dose would have already been
given to these tissues and further irradiation to this region
would be dangerous. The past and future doses of irradiation are

cumulative and together more treatment would inevitably risk irreparable damage to the bladder, rectum, overlying skin, and other surrounding tissues.

Palliative radiotherapy

Cure by surgery is not possible if the cancer has spread beyond the prostate into surrounding tissues, or when there are cancer metastases in areas of bone or other tissues. In these cases radiotherapy can play a very useful role in controlling both local cancer in and around the prostate gland and secondary cancer in other tissues, especially in bone. Secondaries in bone that are causing pain will usually respond to radiotherapy, giving the patient good pain relief.

Surgery and radiotherapy

External radiotherapy using a linear accelerator is often also used in treating those patients who have had radical surgery but in whom there may have been some doubt as to whether all local cancer cells were totally removed. This is the case when the cancer is not confined to the prostate but is found to have spread into nearby tissues or nearby lymph nodes. In such people, surgery followed by radiotherapy should at least theoretically make a cure more likely than would surgery alone, although as yet this has not been proven in regard to prostate cancer.

Case report 4: *Jim, aged 70*

Jim was a 70-year-old retired forester who had become increasingly aware of frequency and difficulty in passing urine over two or three years. After examination by his doctor he was told that his PSA was slightly raised but not high (5.8) but that he had a firm lumpy prostate. He was referred to a urologist who arranged ultrasound and biopsies. When the biopsies were examined by the pathologist, anaplastic cancer cells were found, confirming the diagnosis of an aggressive type of prostate cancer. Although the urologist could feel an area of the prostate that seemed to be fixed (stuck on) to the rectum there was no evidence in bone scans, bone X-rays or chest X-rays of secondaries elsewhere.

The urologist did not think that the prostate would be totally removable by surgery, and in any case Jim, being a long-term smoker, had 'crook lungs' with a productive cough, and some other health problems. An appointment was made for Jim to see a radiotherapist (radiation oncologist). The radiotherapist recommended that the most appropriate treatment for Jim would be by external radiotherapy to the prostate region. This was carried out over six or seven weeks without any serious problems.

Jim's urinary problems improved and his PSA became low (1.0), but it did not fall to zero. Two years later Jim's PSA began to rise, and bone scans showed the presence of secondaries in several bones. Jim felt severe pain in his right hip region, where an X-ray showed a large secondary cancer. This was relieved by radiotherapy to the hip region, and Jim was started on a course of hormone therapy.

Jim lived for another two years without much trouble from his prostate cancer. He died of emphysema and heart failure unrelated to his prostate disease.

10

Hormone treatment

The first evidence that prostate cancers would respond to hormone treatment was when two American doctors, Charles Huggins and Clarence Hodges, discovered that prostate tumours would often become smaller when the patient was given the female hormone stilboestrol. Stilboestrol then became standard treatment for prostate cancer, with most patients gaining benefit and probably some increased life expectancy. However, stilboestrol did not produce a cure in the long term.

Stilboestrol, the female hormone with some anti-male hormone activity, and the more modern derivatives of stilboestrol (called LH-RH analogues) have for years been used as the mainstay for treatment of men with advanced prostate cancer. These have been used when cure by surgery or radiotherapy has not been possible; that is, when the cancer has spread beyond the prostate region with secondaries in bones or other tissues.

Prostate cancer is now known to be testosterone-dependent. That is, without any of the male hormone testosterone, the cancer cells will not grow. Some testosterone needs to be circulating in the blood to keep the cancer cells growing.

Most, but not all, testosterone in men comes from the testes, but the testes can produce testosterone only if they are stimulated by a hormone produced in the brain called gonadotrophic hormone. One way of reducing the growth of prostate cancer therefore is to remove the testes (i.e. castration—a treatment not at all popular with most men). Another way of reducing the effects of testosterone is to find and use an anti-hormone; that is, an anti-testosterone or an anti-gonadotrophin.

More recently, rather than using female-type hormones in treating prostate cancers, a new group of anti-male hormones or male hormone antagonists (anti-androgens) are more commonly used. The most recent of the modern hormones are known as luteinising-hormone releasing-hormone (LH-RH) agonists. These are likely to be both more effective and have fewer side effects than either stilboestrol or the anti-androgens.

There are now a lot of rather different hormone and anti-hormone agents sometimes used to treat secondary or advanced primary prostate cancer. It is now common for the family doctor, or the specialist urologist, or the oncologist, to have a plan of action that is most familiar to them and that in their hands they have found most effective with fewest side effects. However, if the desired response is not achieved, or the patient suffers side effects from any treatment used, a switch can be made to another agent or combination of agents. These agents are known by a number of generic (scientific) names and are produced by different phar-maceutical companies that market them under different trade names. Some of the more commonly used agents are bicalutamide (trade name Casodex), nilatamide (trade name Anandron), gosere-lin acetate (trade name Zoladex; this is given as an implant), or cyproterone acetate (trade name Androcur).

Bicalutamide eliminates the small amount of testosterone that is produced by the adrenal glands after orchidectomy (castration).

Zoladex is a gonadotrophic releasing hormone; that is, it coun-teracts the hormone that stimulates testosterone production.

Androcur is a testosterone antagonist; in effect it reduces the effects of testosterone.

Although cure is not feasible with hormone treatment alone, patients usually benefit with improved passage of urine and relief of bone pain or other symptoms. Sometimes this improvement lasts for a period of only months, but often it lasts for several years. Like any other treatment, there are a number of possible side effects of any hormones. The female hormones especially often cause enlargement of the male breasts and possibly other feminis-ing features. Sometimes the hormones cause nausea and vomiting.

One of the more worrying side effects is a risk of developing a thrombosis (blood clot). Most men given this form of treatment will also lose their sex drive (libido) and usually become impotent.

Some modern hormone and anti-hormone preparations can be taken by mouth daily. Others are given by injection at weekly or less frequent intervals. Some are given by implant under the skin for a long-term, slow-releasing effect. For those men who for one reason or another can't take, or fail to respond to, hormone treatment, removal of the testes (castration) may achieve a similar result, but if hormone treatment has failed it is rather unlikely that there will be further improvement after castration. Although impotence is usual, strangely enough not all men receiving hormone treatment become impotent.

Case report 5: *Russell, aged 47*

Russell was a successful business executive who felt pain in his lower back and passing down his left leg. On performing a digital rectal examination his doctor noticed a lumpiness in Russell's prostate gland, so he arranged to have blood taken for a PSA test. His PSA was a high 9.8. Bone scans and X-rays showed 'hot spots' and calcium deposits (sclerotic lesions) in the lower vertebrae of his backbone, indicative of prostate cancer secondaries. Ultrasound and biopsies of his prostate confirmed the presence of aggressive, anaplastic cancer.

It was explained to Russell that as the cancer had already spread to bones it was not curable by surgery. It was suggested that he should commence hormone treatment with radiotherapy to the secondaries in the vertebrae to try to get most rapid relief of the pain. After further discussion Russell was started on Zoladex by implant, with a short course of bicalutamide tablets. His symptoms improved for five or six months but later recurred. He was then started on Androcur. He felt better for a short time but severe pain in bones troubled him again, so he was treated with bisphosphonate infusion. After three treatments with bisphosphonate infusion he had good pain relief, but four months later severe pain returned. He was then given treatment with strontium 89. He did have further pain relief but a severe fall in platelet count followed—the ability of his blood to clot was seriously reduced—so this treatment was not repeated.

After fourteen months of hormone and medical treatment pain again became severe, so Russell was admitted to a nursing home, where he was given a morphine infusion until he died.

As Russell was relatively young and had a strong family history of prostate cancer—his father and an uncle also died of the disease at a relatively early age—investigations were commenced on Russell's brothers and his son to look for a gene that could be responsible. If such a gene is found his male relatives would be advised to stay under close surveillance so that treatment of any suspected prostate cancer could be commenced at a very early stage.

Case report 6: *Sam, aged 78*

Sam was an age pensioner and had worked in many jobs during his working life. He had been a diabetic for years and had lost a leg from gangrene, but he continued to smoke heavily. He had a chronic and productive cough. He had some frequency and difficulty with passing urine for several years but no other symptoms referable to his prostate.

Sam was found to have a PSA raised to 20.8, suggestive of prostate cancer, but he insisted that apart from getting relief from his urinary difficulties he did not want any further investigation or treatment. A TURP resection was performed under spinal anaesthesia to remove the prostate tissue obstructing his urethra. Cancer cells were found to be present in the tissue removed, but Sam chose not to have any further active investigation or treatment. His urinary difficulties had been relieved for as long as he survived.

Sam died of a stroke three years later, aged 81.

Chemotherapy

Systemic chemotherapy

Modern chemotherapy using anti-cancer drugs has not proven as useful in treating prostate cancer as in treating many other cancers. The main reason is that most anti-cancer agents were not found to be very effective in this cancer when given in doses and concentrations that do not cause toxic side effects. Response to hormones is not only greater and more reliable, but the hormones, especially the anti-androgens, are much less toxic. Avoiding toxicity is especially important in men of this older age group.

Recently, however, trials of the anti-cancer agent mitoxantrone have shown encouraging results in treatment of advanced prostate cancer. Responses have been significant, toxicity is low, and studies have shown improvement of symptoms with improved quality of life.

Regional chemotherapy

The standard method of administering anti-cancer drugs for chemotherapy effectively treats the whole body (systemic chemotherapy). There are presently studies of the use of chemotherapy in greater concentration by infusing the drugs into arteries in the pelvis that supply the prostate with blood. These regional chemotherapy techniques are being investigated, especially in

Germany and Japan, to determine whether the higher concentration of the anti-cancer drugs can achieve a greater effect on the tumour. This is a highly specialised technique, however, and is able to be studied in only a relatively small number of cancer centres. As yet results are uncertain.

Combined integrated treatment

Encouraging results have been shown in studies of combined integrated treatments with hormones, and/or chemotherapy, preceding surgery and/or radiotherapy. In these studies, either hormone treatment or systemic or regional chemotherapy was first used to reduce locally advanced cancers to increase the chance that they would be more curable by the following surgery or radiotherapy. Further studies were made of the use of systemic chemotherapy or hormone treatment as a follow-up treatment after radiotherapy.

Results of these studies have shown that hormone treatment given before surgery or following radiotherapy does improve the outcome in a number of patients, and in many cancer centres this has become one of the standard programs of treatment for locally advanced cancers.

12

Evidence-based medicine

It would be good to think that doctors would always know just what was the right thing to do about every health problem in different people under different circumstances. But the reality is that this is not the case. The evidence is not always there for deciding just what is best for each individual patient under the particular circumstances in which he or she lives. Nowhere in the field of medical practice is the situation more uncertain than in treating men who have, or who might have, a prostate cancer.

In an attempt to solve the uncertainties and sometimes confusion that we know to be true about best medical practice, a new concept has been introduced. It is called 'evidence-based medicine'.

The objective of all doctors has always been to get the best evidence, but in the present days of computerised information, and a variety of approaches in statistical and mathematical analysis and randomised studies, it seemed appropriate to link new scientifically studied and mathematically confirmed clinical information under a group umbrella. This is the approach we call 'evidence-based medicine', as opposed to information based on a one-off experience, a collection of anecdotes, traditionally accepted beliefs, medical folklore, or wishful thinking.

Nowadays most acceptable evidence is usually based on randomised trials. In a randomised trial, all patients with the problem to be studied, in order to discover the best method of care, are invited to take part in a closely observed clinical study. The nature of the trial is explained to them, and if they agree to take part they are randomly allocated into a 'test group'. There are usually two test groups, although in some special studies there may be more. That is, the patients taking part are usually divided into two groups by a lottery-type draw over which none of the interested parties undertaking the studies has any control. (This is why the trial is described as 'randomised'.) Patients in one of the two groups are treated by the best known available standard treatment, and patients in the other group are treated by the new technique under study that it is believed may be an even better method of treatment. Ideally results are recorded 'blind'; that is, by a third party who does not know which patient was given which treatment. Results of the two groups studied are then compared, usually by an appropriate form of statistical analysis, to discover which was the better form of treatment. Such studies are known as controlled randomised studies. Although this is not the only way of finding convincing 'evidence' of best practice, it is usually regarded as the most persuasive. This is because the randomisation means every effort has been made to remove any bias in deciding which patients go into which of the study groups, and 'blind' recording means that how the results are reported should not be influenced by what the researchers expected to happen.

Doctors have always had to make decisions and introduce practices and concepts based on best available evidence, but in the past this evidence was usually gathered from historical evidence or was evidence learned by trial and error. 'Trial and error' is based on the principle of trying not to repeat one's own, or others', mistakes, or of making the fewest possible mistakes. Trial and error has often masqueraded as experience, but one way or another, often by making mistakes, new information was produced and progress was made.

Often traditional or historically accepted practices just 'grew' and became accepted without close analysis or criticism. The dominant medical or surgical teacher may have been skilled in practice but unskilled in critical analysis. Each practitioner's own personal experience was often taken as convincing evidence, without proper analysis or fair comparison with other evidence or different circumstances. This type of a teacher's belief, or of personal experience in a limited practice, is often referred to as 'anecdotal evidence'. And although anecdotal evidence may well be valid, there is no proof that the outcome seen for a particular treatment will be the most consistent if the treatment is used by different practitioners in different circumstances and for different patients. To get that 'proof', practitioners have had to rely on the traditional haphazard methods of trial and error with its inevitable mistakes adding up to 'experience'.

Usually this is not the most appropriate method of making progress. However, there are some notable illustrations of the value of a one-off experience.

Edward Jenner was so convinced that immunisation with the mild disease cowpox would give protection against deadly small-pox that he tested his belief on himself. He injected himself with cowpox and had a mild reaction. He later injected himself with smallpox and, as he had predicted would be the case, did not get the disease. His belief was based on anecdotal observations and historic evidence. There was no scientifically proven information, yet vital medical progress was made. The effectiveness of Jenner's technique was not proven in any randomised trials and in fact has still not been proven by randomised trials.

The approach of Edward Jenner, in using himself as a test case, is still occasionally used in testing strongly held beliefs in other areas of medicine. A report of this type of approach was published in the *Medical Journal of Australia* in 1997 in relation to prostate cancer.

A doctor was diagnosed by biopsies as having prostate cancer. As he believed that there was good evidence that phytoestrogens (plant hormones) could influence the growth of prostate cancer, as do human oestrogens, for the seven days before he underwent radical prostatectomy he treated himself daily with a moderate dose of phytoestrogens. After the surgical removal of the doctor's complete prostate gland, a pathologist was asked to examine the prostate cancer cells and compare their appearance with the appearance of the cancer cells taken in the biopsies prior to any treatment. The pathologist found clear evidence of apoptosis (inbuilt cell death) in the cancer after the treatment, but there was no evidence of apoptosis in the biopsy specimens taken three weeks earlier. This of course was a one-off study, as was the study of Edward Jenner. Although it did not prove anything as convincingly as would a scientifically controlled randomised study, it certainly seemed to indicate that there is a justifiable basis for further such study.

An attempt to determine more scientifically the most likely outcome of different medical practices or treatments has now evolved, especially over the second half of the twentieth century. It is led by medical scientists skilled in statistical analysis and with an aptitude for teasing out patterns in the occurrence of disease. Where possible progress in medical practice is best made in scientifically tested studies where the evidence can be tested and comparisons made and measured against existing best practices. Evidence-based medicine is now becoming the doctor's basic measuring stick for new information and the foundation upon which 'new' and 'old' practices are judged.

This is a great leap forward in the medical profession's ability to make acceptable medical progress more efficient. However, it should not be forgotten that much of our present knowledge, know-how and effective practice was based on a broad range of skills in gathering evidence, and it is still true that not all relevant information can be measured or converted into a computerised model. There is still a need for solutions based on logic, astute observation and close and personal relationships between practitioners and their patients. These relationships and the evidence gained from them must not be lost in the push for mathematically based science. Not all relevant information in medicine can be fed into computer studies to prove mathematically what will achieve the best outcome. Such factors between practitioners and their patients as warmth of the relationship and personal understanding of priorities in social, domestic, spiritual and other circumstances cannot be measured, but they are important in decision-making. Just because they cannot be measured does not mean that they can be ignored or discarded. They do make a difference to outcome as far as people are concerned, and patients are people.

There are so many variations in disease processes, environmental and social situations, human needs, beliefs, emotions, priorities and interpersonal relationships, as well as medical skills, facilities and practices, that it is not always possible to subject even basic information to scientifically designed statistical analysis. This is not to belittle the safer and more acceptable methods of randomised study, but to remind us all that anecdotal or historical evidence or information based on a logically proposed hypothesis might still be the best available evidence, and it must inevitably still play a part in medical thinking and gathering of knowledge.

Evidence based on a logical hypothesis, but not yet ready for a randomised trial, can still be put to the test under a label of a type of scientific study sometimes called a 'pilot study'. The idea and study proposed is usually put to a group of the researcher's 'peers' or well-informed colleagues for comment and approval before being 'trialled' in a small group of well-informed, agreeable and interested patients. If the initial trial is successful, a further and larger group is studied. In this way new ideas can still be tested and new evidence can be gained, under well-organised, closely observed and safe conditions.

Examples exist of important but uncomplicated information gathered without scientific analysis. One obvious example is that there has never been a randomised study to prove that there is a better outcome of treatment of pneumonia with antibiotics than with the best non-antibiotic treatment, as used in pre-antibiotic days. Similarly, anecdotal and historical evidence suggests that surgical removal of an acutely inflamed appendix is likely to achieve a better outcome than the treatment used in pre-anaesthetic days without the intervention of surgery. But in neither case has a controlled randomised study ever been carried out or analysed statistically. Circumstantial evidence and lots of anecdotal information was there, but a scientifically controlled randomised study has never been analysed. Yet who would doubt the value of treating pneumonia with antibiotics or of the surgical removal of an acutely inflamed appendix?

In a more recent context, amputation was the traditional and most effective known treatment for people with advanced cancers in a limb if the cancers were too big to be cut out successfully. Anything less than amputation was known to result in a high risk of the cancer recurring in the same place. Experience in some clinics now indicates that, rather than amputation, in most cases equally satisfactory results can now be achieved by 'shrinking' the cancer with chemotherapy first, and then cutting out the remaining cancer. This has never been 'proven' in a strictly randomised controlled study, and in fact in some clinics amputation is still regarded as the treatment of choice. Ideally the approach should be studied in a properly organised trial, but who would be prepared to ask patients to enter a study in which it depended on the luck of the draw as to whether their limb would be amputated or not? Even if such cooperative patients could be found, would this not be a rather select group of people who would seem to be different from the rest of us?

The human dimension

Statistically valid evidence-based medicine by well-organised randomised studies is the most convincing method of gathering vital information, but the above examples show that it still cannot be used to cover all situations and all aspects of medical practice. Just because some important aspects cannot be converted to a rational mathematical basis that can be tested in a reasonable period of time, it does not mean that they are not important or can be ignored. There are still a number of shortcomings that for the time being continue to elude the mathematicians and statisticians. Historical evidence, clinical experience, patient belief systems, personal and social priorities and needs, and other considerations, still must play an important part in clinical decision-making. The patient must always be regarded as a person first, a person with a health problem, not primarily as a health problem to be solved. The relationship between the doctor and patient must be personal and sacrosanct, based on many unmeasurable and intangible aspects of human emotion as well as knowledge, and applied to the immediate health needs as worked out between patient and doctor, not as dictated by scientific data alone.

Nowhere in medicine are the scientific limitations, variations and uncertainties more evident than in determining what best to do about the possibility of a man having prostate cancer, or even the certainty that he has it. These uncertainties are sometimes further compounded by the doctor having to make a decision as to whether to give advice about, or commence investigation into, the possibility of prostate disease when the patient has no symptoms relevant to prostate disease and has not sought advice about this possibility.

For example, if a 65-year-old man attends his doctor about a cough or a cold or an injury or pain in an arthritic knee, should the doctor remind him that he is now in the age group where he might have a prostate cancer and that a simple PSA test might be a good start to get evidence for this, either positive or negative? Or should the doctor leave him, knowing that if an early cancer were to be found it might be aggressive and might at that stage be curable?

Outcomes of investigation and treatment are still just too unpredictable, but if the matter is raised a decision about what best to do must be made together by the man, possibly with his family or close friends, with best advice given by a friendly, well-informed and unhurried and concerned doctor. Different patients' priorities are often quite different. What will be the right decision for one patient will not necessarily be right for another patient.

Individual judgment and understanding must play important roles, but these are difficult to measure scientifically in dealing with prostate cancer or even the possibility of prostate cancer. As yet evidence-based medicine can play only a limited part in the decision-making process. There are too many individual variables to be taken into consideration. The ultimate decision on whether to investigate, and, if cancer is found, on whether to treat it, must be based on the patient's special and personal priorities and needs, and on the best evidence available of possible outcomes of different courses of action as known to the doctor and potential treatment teams.

13

Controversies in prostate cancer

Nowhere in the field of cancer treatment is there more controversy and confusion than is the case with prostate cancer.

It is often difficult to determine the best or most appropriate treatment for each particular patient. Indeed, it may be difficult to decide whether treatment should be offered at all. This can be an especially difficult decision in men whose prostate cancer is not causing troublesome symptoms. Each of the treatment possibilities has significant side effects that must be considered in deciding how, or whether, to treat cancers that may or may not progress in men mostly of fairly advanced years and often with other health problems. The options of management must be discussed with each patient to try to determine the best treatment for him as an individual with his own life priorities.

The PSA screening test has led to the investigation and diagnosis of prostate cancer in increasing numbers of middle-aged and elderly males. Yet even if a biopsy confirms a diagnosis of cancer, it is estimated that only about one in four or five of those cancers will grow in a malignant fashion and spread to tissues beyond the prostate during the patient's probable life expectancy. There is as yet no way of determining which of those cancers are likely to spread.

Most prostate cancers grow slowly, and even after several years many show no evidence of spread. However, some will spread, to such places as lungs, liver and especially to bones, where they are likely to establish painful secondary growths and lead to the death of the patient.

Appropriate early treatment will cure most patients when the disease is confined to the prostate gland, but all treatments have serious side effects. It is not possible at this stage to determine which patients will benefit from treatment and who might well be left without treatment.

The best indication as to whether a prostate cancer is likely to spread is given by the pathologist after microscopic examination of a biopsy sample or tissue removed during a TURP operation to relieve urinary obstruction (see figure 2.2). If a cancer is small and composed of 'mature' cells, looking most like normal prostate cells, its growth is likely to be very slow and it will probably spread very slowly if at all. Treatment of such a cancer may not be advisable, especially in older men. Those cancers with cells looking most unlike normal prostate cells (called anaplastic) are more likely to invade and spread more rapidly. Early treatment of such cancer should be considered, especially in otherwise healthy younger men with a cancer apparently confined to the prostate gland.

The most unavoidable and distressing side effect of treatment is impotence. This occurs in most treated patients, whether they are treated by total prostatectomy (surgical removal of the whole prostate gland) or by radiation therapy (radiotherapy). Impotence is usual but not inevitable when hormone treatment is used to treat cancers with secondaries, whether by giving female hormones (oestrogens) or by anti-male hormones (anti-androgens), or luteinising-hormone releasing-hormone agonists (LH-RH) or by orchidectomy (castration), or by a combination of these.

Treatment possibilities and considerations

Deciding on the most appropriate method of treatment is complicated by many factors. These include:
- whether the cancer is totally confined to the prostate gland
- the nature of the primary cancer (whether the cancer cells are almost normal or are very abnormal anaplastic cells)

- the nature and location of any secondary cancers (whether it is localised to surrounding lymph nodes, or has spread to bones or other tissues)
- the age and general health of the patient
- the personal lifestyle and life priorities of the patient
- the presently largely indeterminable factor of the likely rate of progression or lack of progression of his cancer.

Although it might be controversial and uncertain as to whether treatment should be recommended, the following are standard treatments that should be considered and discussed between a patient and his medical advisers.

In men who have small cancers that appear to be confined to the prostate gland and who have a life expectancy of more than 10 years, total surgical removal of the prostate gland, possibly with removal of adjacent lymph nodes, should result in cure. There is a certain risk of some complications from this operation but in leading centres with a skilled surgeon and surgical team and an experienced nursing team, for otherwise healthy men the risk of death from the operation is relatively small—less than 1 per cent. Post-operative impotence is highly likely but can be treated effectively in most men.

Alternatively, any obstruction to the flow of urine can be relieved by a TURP operation in which an instrument (resectoscope) is passed into the urethra through the penis and some of the enlarged prostate is cut away. Specimens of the tissue removed are sent for microscopic examination to look for the presence of cancer. The cancer will not be cured by a TURP operation, but there is no physical reason why impotence should result. The risk of death from this procedure is low, less than 0.5 per cent.

Cancer of the prostate will also respond to radiotherapy. This is often used to treat both primary prostatic cancer and a limited number of painful secondary deposits in bone. If the cancer is localised to the prostate gland and surrounding tissues, some patients will be cured by appropriate radiotherapy and the majority will have disease control for the rest of their natural lifespan, although some of these men would have remained well without treatment. Men who have been treated by radiotherapy may have some bladder symptoms and some loss of bowel control, and will probably be impotent. Impotence can now be treated. The cancer treatment might make the men unwell for a time, but there should be no risk of death from the treatment.

Hormone treatment is also used, especially for more wide-spread cancer. Patients with incurable prostate cancer are often given effective palliative relief of symptoms by treatment with one of the oestrogen type or anti-androgen preparations or other hormones, or by bilateral orchidectomy (removal of both testes), or by a combination of these approaches. These treatments give the best relief of symptoms for men with widespread disease. Patients must be informed of the likely side effects of hormone or anti-hormone treatment. Desire for sexual activity will be reduced, and there is likely to be complete impotence. However, as this type of treatment is effective in relieving symptoms in more than 80 per cent of cases, the risk of side effects is usually well justified and acceptable.

Sometimes prostate cancer will respond to treatment with some chemotherapy (cytotoxic) agents. Mitoxantrone is giving very hopeful results in some studies, but chemotherapy is usually used only in patients whose cancer no longer responds to hormone treatment. Hormone treatment is usually more reliable for prostate cancer, more effective, and less toxic, causing fewer unpleasant side effects than cytotoxic agents. Regional chemotherapy (localised intra-arterial chemotherapy that concentrates the drugs to the region of the cancer) is a new, rather more complex and specialised approach, and it is not yet possible to state whether it will be effective either alone or as the first part of a combined, integrated treatment program for locally advanced cancers.

(14)

Complications and palliative care

Urinary problems

Urinary obstruction

If difficulty in or obstruction to passing urine is still present after
treatment, and if it cannot be relieved by a TURP operation
(trans-urethral resection of prostate), it may occasionally be necessary for the surgeon to insert a catheter through the penis and
leave it in place for a prolonged period. The catheter will need to
be changed and replaced at intervals to keep it clean and sterile.
Antibiotics will be given to reduce risk of infection. If the condition continues, it is occasionally necessary to insert a 'supra-pubic'
catheter. This is a catheter placed surgically into the bladder
through a small opening in the lower abdomen. These catheters
drain continuously, or a special valve may be used so they drain
intermittently, into a special plastic bag, usually strapped onto one
of the thighs. The bag is emptied about twice daily, morning and
evening.

Urinary incontinence

After prostatectomy all men lose control of their urine for a period
of between two or three weeks to several weeks. Initially a catheter
is left in place to drain into a plastic bag, as described above.
This can be followed by fitting a plastic sheath rather like a

condom over the penis; this drains into a plastic bag strapped to the thigh. This plastic bag is emptied as necessary, usually twice daily.

The patient is taught to carry out exercises to strengthen the pelvic muscles that control urine flow, and eventually urinary control should return. Subsequently, however, the patient may sometimes not have complete control and he may choose to wear a small pad in his underpants to absorb any dribble that might occur, especially at times of mental or physical stress or tiredness, or when he has a full bladder.

Impotence

Impotence is common after radical prostatectomy, radiotherapy, and any form of hormone treatment. Men must be warned of this risk, especially as some men with cancer localised to the prostate gland may live untroubled by the cancer for years. Impotence after prostatectomy occurs because important nerves supplying the penis have to be cut in the operation and the rich network of blood vessels that engorge the penis with blood to produce an erection will have been damaged in the operation.

The problem of impotence after prostatectomy can usually be overcome by one of several techniques, as discussed below.

In some men an alternative way to achieve sexual satisfaction may be oral sex with a cooperative partner. This can often be achieved with or without a full erection or, in some men, even without an erection at all.

All these possibilities can be discussed freely with the urologist or an experienced family doctor or perhaps even better with a specialist sex therapist. There is no need for embarrassment—they have heard it all before.

Penile prostheses

Before effective drugs became available to help stimulate an erection, some surgeons performed a surgical operation in which the non-functioning erectile tissue was removed and an inflatable prosthesis was inserted into the penis. A small fluid-filled bag was placed under the skin of the lower abdomen; this could be pressed to inflate the prosthesis, resulting in an erection.

This is a significant surgical procedure to perform on older men whose need for erection may or may not be important to them. For some the operation is successful and much appreciated, but not all such operations are successful. A good deal of discussion and counselling is advisable before a decision is made to have this procedure. Nowadays non-surgical treatments are usually preferred, at least on a trial basis, before deciding on an implant.

Prostaglandins

The most reliable treatment for impotence at this stage is for the patient to learn to give himself injections of a hormone (prostaglandin) into the penis.

The injection will usually be followed by penile erection, and in about 10 minutes or so sexual intercourse can be performed with orgasm but without ejaculation. The patient will need to find out for himself, by trial, exactly what dose is best for him to inject into his penis to obtain a satisfactory erection. It is usually advisable to start using a small dose at first, perhaps 5 or 10 micrograms (0.5 or 1.0 millilitres). Depending on the response of the penis in achieving a satisfactory erection and the time taken for the penis to return to its normal non-erection resting state, the man may increase or even decrease the amount injected on future occasions. The patient should report his success or lack of success to his doctor, who can help in deciding whether a change in technique or dose injected is advisable.

Men need to be reminded that injection alone will probably not achieve a satisfactory erection. First the man must learn the technique of squeezing the base of the penis for a few minutes during and after the injection to help retain the injected fluid in the penis itself, and this must be followed by a certain amount of normal sexual stimulation or foreplay to provide the right stimulus for full erection. The patient is advised not to have a penile injection more than twice in any week, as scarring and damage to the penis can result from too-frequent injections.

Various preparations of prostaglandins are available with a variety of trade names.

Viagra

At least in some men, probably the majority, the erection stimulation drug Viagra can be effective in helping achieve a satisfactory erection after prostatectomy. In most men some of the nerves important in causing an erection will have escaped damage during surgery, but in others the damage may have been complete and irreversible. It is still uncertain just how reliable and effective Viagra will be in helping men who have had such radical surgery or radical radiotherapy to treat prostate cancer.

As with prostaglandins, the dose needed to achieve a satisfactory erection must be discovered by the patient, with the doctor advising. After the man has tried a small dose (perhaps a 50-milligram tablet first) and discussed with his doctor his first experience with it, he and his doctor can begin to work out the dose required.

Viagra must be taken about one hour before the expected intercourse, as it takes this time to achieve its maximal response. Again, some form of sexual stimulation, with foreplay or whatever, is needed to complement the effect of the drug.

In all men some side effects of Viagra are likely. The most common is some flushing of the face, but a more serious drop in blood pressure is also likely. Viagra should not be taken with alcohol, as the combination of alcohol and Viagra can be dangerous. In some men the fall in blood pressure can be dangerous, and for these men Viagra must be avoided. This is especially so in men who take nitrite medications for a heart condition. These men should never take Viagra. Some other technique of achieving an erection may be tried, but Viagra must be avoided. Viagra may be unsafe for any elderly man with a heart condition.

Another drawback to the use of Viagra is its cost. It is an expensive drug and in Australia (year 2000 prices) it costs about 20 dollars for each tablet.

Muse

A newer erection-stimulating agent marketed as Muse has recently become available, and this may have advantages over both prostaglandin injections and Viagra.

Muse is a medication that is inserted into the urethra at the end of the penis. It is inserted by an applicator through the opening in the end of the penis; the applicator is then withdrawn. This avoids the painful injection by a needle into the penis needed for prostaglandins, although it is not as reliable in achieving an erection as penile injections.

Because it acts locally, Muse also avoids the general flushing and other possible side effects of Viagra. It is also quicker in its action than Viagra, taking only about 10 minutes to act. The man will still need some form of sexual stimulation to fully achieve the effect of Muse.

One of the big drawbacks of Muse is its cost. At present (year 2000) prices in Australia, one injection of Muse costs about 70 dollars; that is, it costs about 70 dollars per use.

Pain

In the early post-operative stages analgesics such as paracetamol may be required from time to time to relieve pain, but aspirin is not recommended as it can cause bleeding. Later aspirin can be a very useful drug in men of this age group. Not only does it relieve pain, but it also reduces risk of clotting in the legs and elsewhere; it also reduces risk of coronary artery disease and stroke. It may also reduce of risk of some other health problems, for example bowel cancer.

For more severe pain, as for example from bone secondaries, the best treatment is to treat the secondaries in the bone. This is usually by radiotherapy if only one or two bones are affected, or by hormone treatment if the bone pain is widespread with several secondaries. Bone fractures will require orthopaedic treatment, possibly by surgical plating or pinning.

Results with the use of bisphosphonates or strontium 89 in relieving pain from bone secondaries have been so encouraging that these agents are now more or less standard treatment for bone pain in modern oncology units. Details of their use are discussed in chapter 15.

If bone pain is severe and cannot otherwise be controlled, it might be necessary to use stronger pain-relieving drugs like morphine or pethidine.

Social, psychological and spiritual help

People being treated for cancer, especially an advanced or incurable cancer, will usually require more help and support than just that provided by a busy surgeon, radiotherapist or medical oncologist, or even the family doctor. The family doctor should, however, be a regular member of, or at least in regular contact with, the treatment team.

Depending upon the individual patient's family support, home, and domestic, social, work, business or financial circumstances, there will be different needs. It is important for the treatment team to become aware of the needs of each patient, and usually to enlist support of family members as well as a social worker, perhaps a psychologist, member of the clergy, or even, if emotional disturbance is severe, a psychiatrist. Eventually help of a palliative care specialist may be needed.

Long-term follow-up care

After the initial problems associated with treatment have been settled, a regular follow-up pattern of management and support should be planned, usually with the family doctor. It is best if the family doctor keeps in regular contact and consultation with the specialist team as necessary. One important need is to help take care of any residual problems such as impotence, as already discussed.

An important follow-up procedure after curative surgery or radiotherapy is for subsequent PSA studies to be carried out.

These are to determine whether the cancer has been cured. If the PSA levels remain very low the patient can be virtually assured of cure. If the PSA level rises again, or if there is other evidence of residual cancer, then further treatment, possibly with hormones or radiotherapy, might be indicated.

15

Secondary (metastatic) prostate cancer

In some men (a very small minority), a prostate cancer may have spread to other parts of the body before the patient has been troubled by any problem with the prostate or urinary flow. The first indication of a problem may be when a cancer is found in a bone or some other tissue. These secondary cancers are due to prostate cancer cells that found their way to other parts of the body before the man had any indication that he had anything wrong with his prostate.

In other men, when a cancer has been found in the prostate the doctor will arrange tests to find out if there is any evidence of the cancer in bones or any other tissue or organ away from the prostate. The most common such tests are a chest X-ray, bone scan, and bone X-rays.

Before any decision can be made about the most appropriate treatment, the treatment team must know as best they can what the extent of the cancer is. They need to know whether the cancer is in the prostate and in the prostate only, or in the prostate and possibly in tissues around the prostate, or in the prostate and lymph nodes near the prostate, or in bones or other tissues or organs away from the prostate.

Occasionally later tests may show evidence of cancer spread, months or years after the cancer had apparently been cured by surgery or radiotherapy. Sometimes the cancer spread may first show up when it causes pain or other symptoms in a bone or other part of the body. In these cases the cancer cells must have got there as a small spot called a micrometastasis before the prostatectomy or radiation therapy had been carried out. The tiny micrometastasis, too small to detect at the time, has remained dormant or has grown only very slowly, taking months or years to get to a size big enough to show up.

It is especially to help identify any such patient that close follow-up testing is required after radical treatment of prostate cancer, whether the treatment was by operation or by radiation therapy or both. If evidence of spread can be detected before it has caused serious trouble, it is more likely that a treatment to control the site of trouble can be effective. It is much more difficult if it is left for serious problems to occur, such as possibly a painful or broken bone.

PSA

There are a few simple and easily available tests in long-term follow-up observations. The first of these is a digital examination of the rectum and adjacent tissues in what was previously the place of the prostate. The second is a chest X-ray, simply because it is easily arranged and may also be useful in a general health check of the patient. The most important, however, is regular PSA testing. Some doctors believe that this is the single most important use of the PSA test.

If, after initial cancer treatment, the PSA falls to zero or close to zero (less than 0.2 millimols per litre), this is a good indication that the treatment was effective and the cancer was totally exterminated. Occasionally, however, the PSA level starts to creep up again in a man who was thought to have been cured. If this happens it is an indication that some cancer cells have survived and have started to grow again in some part of the body.

Under the circumstance of a rising PSA in a man who is otherwise reasonably fit and well, a search is likely to be recommended to the patient to find the site or sites of the recurrent or secondary cancer, so that any appropriate advice or treatment can be planned.

Bone scan, bone X-rays and chest X-rays

Given the rising PSA, the most useful single further test is likely to be a bone scan. The bone scan should indicate in which bones and in what parts of the bones increased activity, caused by growth of cancer cells, is taking place.

If the bone scan shows only one or two 'hot spots', X-rays will be arranged to try to get further information about the extent of the cancer and the damage that it is causing in the bone or bones. Secondary prostate cancer in bones usually accumulates calcium and therefore the secondaries are commonly seen as white or 'sclerotic' round deposits in the bone X-rays (see figure 2.3). Knowing the extent of the problem will allow consideration of what treatment, possibly with radiotherapy, can be arranged, particularly if pain or other symptoms are present.

If bone scans show many 'hot spots' in the bones, further treatment is usually directed to the whole body to affect cancer cells wherever they may be. This usually means arranging some form of anti-cancer hormone treatment, as discussed in chapter 10. If one or two spots in particular are causing pain, then those spots may be treated with radiotherapy.

Treatment of metastases

If 'hot spots' in bone scans indicate that secondaries are present but they are not causing pain, a decision will need to be made as to whether or not the patient would benefit from treatment. If the patient is elderly and not well and the secondaries are small in size and in a position not likely to cause an immediate problem, it may be best simply to repeat the scans in some months' time to see if they change significantly. For most patients, however, some form of treatment is usually advisable. Most men, if not already having hormone treatment, would be advised to have a hormone treatment program.

If only two or three 'hot spots' are seen and especially if they are in a position likely to cause serious trouble, such as in a backbone (vertebra) near the spinal cord or in a major weight-bearing bone likely to fracture, treatment with radiation therapy is likely to retard further growth of any radiation-treated metastasis. If there are many 'hot spots', irradiation is best administered to those two or three or four most in danger of causing serious trouble or those already causing pain. Radiation therapy cannot be safely given to more than a limited number of secondaries.

If an important bone, especially a weight-bearing bone such as the femur (the large long bone in the thigh and hip), has fractured, then the help of a skilled orthopaedic specialist will be needed. The bone may need to be repaired or supported by a metal nail or plate.

Bisphosphonates

It has recently been found that a group of drugs called bisphosphonates can help bones resist destruction by some secondary cancers. The bisphosphonates become incorporated in the weakened area of bone, restoring some strength to the bone and helping it resist further destruction.

For secondaries from prostate cancer it is uncertain whether bisphosphonates act to help bones resist invasion and bone destruction by prostate cancer cells (as they do in breast cancer, for example), but they do relieve bone pain in many patients with prostatic secondary cancer in bone.

For bisphosphonate treatment the patient needs to attend his hospital or oncology unit for a couple of hours. There, a slow drip of fluid containing the drug is infused into a vein. The patient simply sits or lies comfortably during the procedure, reading a book or perhaps watching television. The treatment should not worry him or cause side effects. It can be repeated at about monthly intervals if necessary.

One of the available bisphosphonates (disodium pamidronate) is traded as Aredia.

Strontium 89

Another new agent found to help men with metastatic cancer in bones is strontium 89. This is a radioactive isotope of an element that becomes incorporated in bones, as does calcium. Strontium 89 especially becomes incorporated in bone tissue being destroyed by cancer cells. The radiation from the strontium 89 destroys cancer cells in the bone and gives pain relief. The small dose of beta irradiation does not penetrate far into tissues and so is not dangerous to other parts of the body or to anyone else nearby.

As strontium 89 does risk certain side effects it is usually not repeated in less than three months and then only if there has been a complete recovery from any adverse effect on bone marrow (especially a fall in blood platelets) or any other side effect.

Studies continue, but there is some evidence that these new agents, the bisphosphonates and strontium 89, may help protect bones from further secondary invasion of cancer cells.

Other anti-cancer drugs

The standard anti-cancer chemotherapy drugs that are commonly effective against other types of cancer are usually not of great help in treating prostate cancer. The anti-cancer drug mitoxantrone might be proving an exception. In general, treatment with hormones is much more likely to be effective and has less risk of distressing or potentially debilitating side effects.

Pain-relieving drugs and palliative care

Other than hormone management, bisphosphonates or strontium 89, the standard treatment of pain due to metastatic prostate cancer is the use of pain-relieving drugs, as previously discussed. Usually the less powerful drugs like paracetamol (Panadol, Tylenol) are used first, then, as necessary, stronger agents like codeine, then later pethidine or morphine, may be required. Codeine and morphine are both likely to cause constipation that may then require treatment.

In advanced cases of cancer when the patient is experiencing severe distress, the care of a team skilled in palliative care can be a blessing. These caring medical, nursing and paramedical people are skilled at keeping their patients as comfortable as possible, sometimes in the surroundings of their own homes. If necessary patients will be cared for in a special nursing home or a hospice, whatever will give the individual patient the best physical and psychological relief in an environment as stress-free and comfortable as possible.

16

The relationship between the patient and his doctors

Nowhere in the field of medical practice are good personal relationships, trust and understanding more important than between each patient with cancer and his or her medical advisers. Prostate cancer stands out as having special need for a good relationship because of the uncertainties over what is best for the patient.

There is no simple answer, and each man's special needs and priorities and his family and social relationships and circumstances are all important in the decision-making. Added to this need is the common reluctance of men with these sorts of personal problems, which they have usually regarded as especially private and confidential, to express their inner thoughts and anxieties to someone who will take time to talk it over with them.

By the time men reach the age of having need for advice about prostate matters, most will know a family doctor in whom they have trust and confidence. If not they should seek one, perhaps on the recommendation of a friend or friends who have had similar problems.

After comfortable, unhurried, and mutually thoughtful and honest discussion with his family doctor about his problems, and at least on one occasion with his wife, partner or other close family member or friend present, arrangements will often be made for consultation with a specialist.

The specialist is unlikely to be an old family friend, as the family doctor may well be, but it is equally important for the family doctor to arrange referral of the patient to a skilled but compassionate; supportive and understanding specialist who is prepared to listen to the patient's anxieties and take time to answer his many asked or unasked questions. The specialist should be chosen because he or she has special skills, facilities and expertise, and is readily available to communicate comfortably with an anxious, troubled and confused man and his family. This is not the occasion for the family doctor to arrange consultation with a specialist predominantly because he or she was an old school mate or one who had just come back from overseas with good training and needs support.

Certainly the specialist must have the appropriate skills and facilities and must be up-to-date with the latest information, but over and above this it is most important for the specialist to be able to communicate and explain, to be ready to answer questions freely and in an unhurried atmosphere, and to be readily accessible, possibly by telephone, if or when problems or questions arise. Discussions about the most appropriate treatment should not sound like an edict from above but should be mutually considered and arranged, having taken into account many factors special to the individual patient. The specialist must also appreciate that no matter how clearly he or she has explained everything to the patient, it is unlikely that the patient will be able to take it all in in one visit. One or more further visits are almost essential for probably every patient, if not to the specialist then at least to the well-informed family doctor.

The relationship between specialist and patient will probably be prolonged over several months or years. In fact there should be a close three-way relationship with good understanding and communication between specialist, family doctor and patient.

17

Future directions

The future for the cancer sufferer is a mixture of hope and caution.

Diet and lifestyle

To avoid cancers in general, people should be encouraged to accept some changes to the typical Western lifestyle. These changes include a reduction of animal fats in the diet and a reduced consumption of artificial chemical preservatives and other chemical additives and contaminants in their food, in favour of food that provides a greater intake of fibre, with more fresh fruits and vegetables, nuts, grains and protective legumes. There should be a policy of avoiding sunburn or excessive ultraviolet irradiation, moderation in the use of alcohol, and, especially, no smoking.

There will continue to be advances based on epidemiological information, such as a better understanding of the protective qualities of high-fibre diets and the apparent protective qualities of diets high in other possible protective agents (such as the naturally occurring plant hormones—the phytoestrogens—and lycopene). These particularly apply in reducing the risk of prostate cancer in men, breast cancer in women, and bowel cancer in both sexes.

Learning from alternative and naturopathic practices

More will be learned from alternative medicine and naturopathic practices as well as from drawing upon traditions and practices of ancient and 'undeveloped' communities. However, care must be taken to analyse such practices properly and not to allow wishful thinking, emotion or 'fashion' to cloud scientific and clinical judgment.

It must be appreciated that, before any new medication can be safely recommended, extensive tests and studies are necessary to be sure that the agent does not have serious side effects or toxic properties. Just because a substance is 'natural' or extracted from plants does not mean that it is safe to use. Cancer-causing products like tobacco and betel nut are 'naturally grown' plant products, as are the poison strychnine and many other toxic and poisonous substances.

Improved cancer screening

Another measure of increasing importance is regular screening of people at special risk for certain types of cancer, including prostate cancer, so that any early signs can be detected and treated before an advanced cancer develops.

It is anticipated that improved, more accurate and simpler screening measures will become available in the future. These may include simple blood screening tests for cancer antibodies or other tumour markers to indicate the presence of early cancer at a more curable stage and before symptoms have developed.

A great need in the case of prostate cancer is for a refined screening test to detect which people with a raised PSA have prostate cancer and which have some other non-malignant prostate trouble. Not only does the present PSA screening identify some men who do not have cancer, it also misses some men with prostate cancer who do not have elevated PSA levels. A more accurate test of prostate cancer is still sought. A new test of activity (methylation) of a prostate oncogene is hopeful.

However, the greatest practical need is for a test to indicate just which prostate cancers are likely to behave in an aggressively malignant fashion. A way is needed to distinguish between cancers that will continue to grow and invade surrounding tissues and spread to other places, and cancers that are likely to lie dormant for many years without becoming life-threatening during the patient's expected lifetime (the so-called 'latent' prostate cancers). Such a test, if found to be reliable, might avoid the need for aggressive treatment or even the need for treatment at all in possibly the majority of patients detected with cancer cells in their prostate gland.

Improved early detection, diagnostic and treatment techniques

Present techniques of detection, diagnosis and management have been described in earlier chapters. Improvements and newer techniques in all these areas are inevitable. Improved diagnostic measures will help establish more certain and more accurate diagnosis at an earlier stage. Already improvements in CT (computerised tomography) scanning and other organ imaging techniques have made considerable advances for some cancers, and further advances are assured. Magnetic resonance imaging (MRI) has added to these improved diagnostic and imaging methods.

It is anticipated that within a few years the relatively new method of organ imaging called PET (positron emission tomography) might make an even greater impact than CT and MRI scanning. PET scans give additional information about activity, composition and survival of tumour cells, as well as detecting secondary cancer cells at an earlier stage than has been possible in the past.

A PET scan involves no more discomfort or disturbance than having a CT scan. First an injection of a glucose material is given. About 50 minutes later the patient lies on a scanning table in a room where a scanner moves over and around him for about an hour. Apart from the needle prick it is quite painless.

Other studies are now being conducted using a newer related test called magnetic resonance scanning (MRS). These studies are carried out on prostate cancer cells taken by biopsy. The tests are carried out in especially equipped research laboratories where it is hoped that results will indicate whether the cancer cells are aggressive and dangerous or likely to remain relatively quiescent and pose little risk to life. They may also be able to indicate which hormones or which anti-cancer drugs are most likely to be effective against the particular cancer cells involved.

Of the newer techniques for determining those prostate cancers likely to behave aggressively and those likely to remain as 'latent' cancer without being life-threatening, the most hopeful lines of investigation might be with the MRS and the PET scan techniques. These tests are based on the physiological and biochemical activity of cancer cells, and this could well be a more hopeful approach to getting information about the cancer cell activity than the anatomical size, shape, position and boundaries as shown by CT, MRI and other studies.

Improved pathology techniques such as fine-needle aspiration cytology (using a syringe and needle to suck out cells for immediate examination) and frozen section techniques (see chapter 8) have allowed major progress in establishing early detection and the nature of early tumours. These instruments and their application will also undoubtedly continue to be improved.

Improved chemotherapy

There is progress in improved treatment with more effective and more specific anti-cancer drugs. In particular, there is improved knowledge of how best to use anti-cancer drugs in appropriate combinations and treatment schedules that achieve increased anti-tumour results with a reduced risk of toxicity and fewer or less severe unwanted side effects.

New and more effective anti-cancer agents like the taxanes are constantly being tested in treating different cancers and some are added to the range of available anti-cancer drugs. Many drugs are being made safer and more effective with the increasing availability of agents that protect bone marrow and other body tissues from harmful side effects. New laboratory testing methods will also give information as to which treatment methods and which anti–cancer agents are likely to be of greatest benefit in treating each individual cancer.

Although at this stage these studies are more applicable to other types of cancer in younger people, eventually there may well be methods of screening for and determining more specific anti–cancer treatments for men with prostate cancer.

Angiostatic and angiotoxic agents

A new and hopeful avenue of further research in cancer treatment uses angiostatic and angiotoxic agents. These have the potential to destroy cancers by destroying the new fragile blood vessels the cancers depend upon for their essential blood supply.

Apoptosis-promoting anti-cancer agents

Another new approach in anti–cancer treatment is the search for agents to promote apoptosis in cancer cells.

Normal tissue cells have a limited lifespan. They self–destruct after an apparently inbuilt period of time when they are no longer needed and have been replaced by new cells. This process is called apoptosis.

Cancer cells have lost the ability to self–destruct, but there is some evidence that it may be possible to restore the self–destructive property to cancer cells, possibly by administration of certain biological agents. One of the more interesting studies of this type is being made in relation to certain naturally occurring phytoestrogens (plant hormones) or related compounds. Studies suggest that under some circumstances phytoestrogens appear to have the ability to restore apoptosis properties to prostate cancer cells.

Improvements in radiotherapy

Treatment by radiotherapy is also being constantly improved, with different types of radiation emission and different treatment schedules integrated with anti–cancer drugs or hormones for more effective treatment. Studies continue, especially with brachytherapy, which administers the irradiation directly to the cancer by implantation of radioactive materials into the cancer.

Integrated treatments

It does not seem that surgery for the eradication of cancers generally will advance greatly over present techniques. There are a few possible exceptions, such as organ replacement (not likely to be applicable to prostate surgery) or the use of regional tissue perfusion techniques. However, there is a need for an increasing role for better organised and better planned, combined integrated treatment schedules to improve the treatment of advanced cancers.

In these treatment schedules chemotherapy, radiotherapy and surgery are used more effectively in combined approaches that are planned from the outset. Further studies are under way into the use of surgical measures and radiologically placed intra-arterial catheter techniques. In this a fine catheter is placed, under X-ray control by a radiologist, into an artery supplying blood to the cancer. This is intended to distribute, more selectively, anti-cancer agents in greater concentration to the region of a tumour. Together with PET scan imaging to monitor progress, it is anticipated that in the future treatment will be directed more selectively to parts of the body where it is needed.

Heat therapy

Another treatment, not well exploited as yet, makes use of the known increased susceptibility of cancer cells to heat. Studies of the application of heat to eradicate tumour cells selectively, possibly in combination with anti-cancer drugs, may improve treatment techniques for certain types of cancer. However, as yet there is no evidence that this will apply to prostate cancer in the immediate future.

One possible avenue of using heat to achieve more effective treatment might be in conjunction with regional chemotherapy and/or regional immunotherapy. In treating some other advanced localised cancers with closed-circuit perfusion chemotherapy using heart–lung pump equipment, which confines the chemo-therapy agent to the region of the cancer, cancers have been found to be more responsive when the anti-cancer agents have been perfused in greater concentration and in a heated perfusion circuit. That is, the concentrated anti-cancer drugs have been more effective when they are applied to the cancer at an increased temperature.

Cryosurgery

As opposed to heat, extreme cold by freezing is also used in treat-ment of some cancers. Freezing with subsequent thawing destroys cells, including cancer cells.

At present these techniques are used most often in treating cancers in the liver. Many technical difficulties need to be solved before such techniques could be applied to prostate cancers in the pelvis.

Electrolysis

Another approach being investigated as a possible technique for destroying cancer cells is the application of electrolysis—electric currents—by means of probes inserted into the tumour region.

At this stage the technique is being studied for its potential in destroying cancer masses in the liver, but if it is found to be successful there, its application in treating other localised cancers such as in the prostate is likely to follow.

Immunotherapy

A lot of people, including many cancer experts, believe that the greatest hope for cancer treatment in general in the future is in the field of immunotherapy.

Cancers are often thought to be due to a deficiency in the body's immune defence system. Whereas abnormal cells are usually recognised and eradicated by the body's natural immune defences, in the cancer patient the abnormal cells have continued to survive and multiply. There is a great deal of supportive evidence for this 'immune surveillance theory', but one piece of evidence lies in the fact that very occasionally a really advanced and aggressive type of cancer will suddenly and spontaneously disappear without trace for no apparent reason. Such self-healing is all too rare, but there have been some well-documented reports of it in the medical and scientific literature. This suggests that somehow the body's natural defence mechanisms have taken charge again.

A great deal of work has been carried out in leading hospitals, cancer institutes and other institutions, in the search for greater knowledge and application of the immunological defence mechanisms. There is hope that specific immunological tumour markers—features of cancer cells that can be recognised by special immune tests—will reveal evidence of the presence of certain cancers very early and before they can otherwise be detected clinically. There is hope too not only that tumour antibodies may reveal early evidence of cancer but also that they may be used in treatment, either in a direct attack upon cancer cells or by carrying cytotoxic chemical agents specifically to the cancer cells. There is hope that a more reliable means of stimulating the immune defence system to eradicate cancer cells will emerge from these studies.

Preparations of monoclonal antibodies are now available for some tumours, and treatments based on their use are under study, but as yet these techniques do not seem to apply to prostate cancer. Studies with products of the immune defence system such as interferon and the interleukins have not yet had the impact originally expected and as yet they have no application to prostate cancer.

Recent research indicates that another product of the immune system, tumour necrosis factor (TNF), may have more practical value for some cancers, especially when used in combination with other anti-cancer agents, in localised intra-arterial regional chemotherapy programs.

Genetic engineering

New techniques of molecular DNA biology offer a different approach in combating cancer. It may soon be possible to change the structure of DNA in cells and thus change the nature of actually or potentially malignant cells into cells without the propensity for malignant growth.

The new science of genetic engineering also has potential for changing the basic nature of cells to prevent cancer developing, or to change the nature of malignant cells. Although there have been some small trials of gene therapy, unfortunately there is as yet no evidence that an application of these techniques will solve present problems of prostate cancer.

Prevention of metastases

Chemical agents like the bisphosphonates appear to have protective qualities in prevention of certain bone secondaries, and further studies into their use have created much interest. It may be that these substances have the ability to promote apoptosis in cells forming secondary cancers in bone.

New work in the use of strontium 89 has also stimulated more studies in the ability of this and similar agents to protect against metastases.

Improved palliative care

For those people with advanced cancer and in great discomfort or pain, methods of relieving the suffering with understanding counsel and comfort are now better understood. Such measures are now more readily available, and there is now little need for patients to suffer greatly from pain or other distressing symptoms of cancer. Palliative care specialist units are constantly improving the care and relief of distress of patients with cancer, including men with advanced prostate cancer.

Hope for the future

As for any health problem, and especially cancer, the greatest hope for the future lies in prevention. The best treatment for cancer is to do everything you can not to get one.

With increasing information and comparison of those men and communities with high and low incidence of this cancer, there are now exciting prospects of reducing the incidence of prostate cancer in men of Western communities. The best prospects for this appear to lie either in dietary changes or in adding missing ingredients to Western diets, or possibly a combination of these approaches.

However, for those with serious but not terminal disease, hope must be maintained. The probability or possibility of cure is now available for increasing numbers of patients with cancer.

Even for patients now considered to have incurable disease, worthwhile palliation is now available with the hope that, for some, further improvement in treatment methods with every prospect of cure may be around the corner.

Research teams are constantly making progress, and well-conducted research must be supported. Not every research project will be a winner, but some will make new and important discoveries.

18

Conclusions

Prostate cancer is the most commonly diagnosed internal cancer in Western men of modern times. This is due to a number of factors. Greater numbers of men are now living to old age. Modern diagnostic techniques mean prostate cancer is detected earlier than used to be the case. There was also an increase in incidence of prostate cancer in men of Western societies during the twentieth century.

Improved methods of treatment for men with this cancer are also now available, but they all have serious side effects, most often leaving treated patients impotent.

For the present, the greatest need in prostate cancer is not so much in achieving better diagnosis or treatment, but in determining which patients with a diagnosis of localised prostate cancer should have treatment at all. In a large number of men, probably the majority, the cancer is unlikely to behave aggressively and spread. In many of these men it is likely to lie dormant as a 'latent' cancer without causing the patient any great trouble, or possibly causing no trouble at all, during his otherwise expected lifetime. However, if the cancer is one of the apparent minority that will behave aggressively and spread, if it is not stopped it can lead to a most distressing, painful, and miserable mode of death for the patient.

Which is the most appropriate treatment, or whether to have any treatment at all, or indeed whether to initiate screening or diagnostic tests in men who have no symptoms, presents a very real series of dilemmas for the patient and his doctors. Some doctors, including some specialists and anti-cancer organisations, take the view that it is better not to do the PSA screening test in otherwise fit men without symptoms. Their attitude is that until there is a method of determining which cancers will progress and become life-threatening, it is kinder to leave the patient living comfortably and happily rather than tell him he has a cancer but there is no way of being sure whether or not it should be treated. This is especially so as any form of treatment will leave him with side effects, in particular a high risk of becoming impotent.

For most younger men who are otherwise in good health and in whom there is evidence that a cancer is localised only to the prostate gland, and therefore most probably curable by surgery, and especially if it contains anaplastic or aggressive cancer cells, surgical removal is likely to be the preferred option of treatment. This is particularly so if there is any indication of the cancer enlarging or if increasing PSA levels suggest increasing growth and activity.

Fortunately there are now ways of restoring the ability for sexual activity in most men made impotent by surgery.

For older and less fit men, and especially when there is a real doubt about the total removability of the cancer and whether the cancer is progressing, radiotherapy is likely to be the preferred treatment. Alternatively, and especially in older or unfit men without troublesome symptoms, the most appropriate option might be not to have any active treatment until, if or when troublesome symptoms arise.

At present perhaps the most positive new approach is to try to avoid the problem arising in the first place. With our present state of knowledge, the most hopeful avenue for prevention of prostate cancer in men of Western societies appears to be to adopt a diet, and more importantly to encourage young children to adopt diets, more like those in countries and societies where prostate cancer is uncommon. This suggests that men of Western societies should eat predominantly vegetarian diets with larger quantities of soy, including soy milk, and/or other legumes, nuts and grains. New studies of possible preventive effects of lycopene, the natural red colouring in tomatoes, suggest that increased quantities of tomato preparations should be included in the average diet. Alternatively, similar results might be achieved by keeping basically to Western diets but with more fruits and vegetables, and especially tomato preparations, and with a reduced content of animal fat. A more regular intake of lycopene, as in foods containing cooked tomatoes, might also help prevent prostate cancer. Perhaps this modified diet might be further improved by supplementing it with an occasional tomato-rich pizza and a concentrated isoflavone tablet daily.

Making a final decision about treatment

The greatest difficulty in prostate cancer is in making a decision about treatment for a man with a localised and potentially curable cancer.

Described in this book are the active treatments that are available and might be effective in treating and possibly curing prostate cancer, but making the right choice of treatment or no treatment remains difficult for both the patient and his medical advisers. The major decision for a man with no symptoms caused by the cancer is in deciding whether or not any treatment is justified, given only one in four or five prostate cancers is likely to become aggressive and life-threatening during the man's likely period of life expectancy. The decision to treat or not to treat can only be made after close and personal discussion between the patient, his closest family or friends and his medical advisers, after all circumstances and life priorities have been considered.

As a general rule I would recommend treatment by radical surgery or alternatively combined radiotherapy for a younger man with a proven cancer that is apparently localised to the prostate gland but which is possibly showing evidence of anaplasia or invasive characteristics, especially if the patient has a rising PSA. This advice applies provided the man has an otherwise good life expectancy of at least ten years for surgery or five years for radiotherapy.

For an older man with a similar cancer but otherwise with a life expectancy of less than ten years, if the cancer is treated at all other than to relieve urinary obstruction I would recommend radiotherapy.

It is for the men between these two extremes with an apparently localised cancer that a firm recommendation is difficult. A final choice must be made by the patient and those close to him, having considered his life priorities.

Decisions are less difficult in recommending treatment for a man with prostate cancer that has locally spread beyond the prostate gland but apparently not to more distant sites. Radical surgery is not likely to cure the cancer, but local radiotherapy may still achieve a cure. A TURP operation may be appropriate to relieve obstruction to urine flow.

For a man with widespread secondary cancer, although many options of hormone treatment have been described, or possibly chemotherapy, or radiotherapy to a limited number of troublesome secondaries, it is usually not difficult to make an appropriate decision, at least on a trial basis.

An elderly man with no symptoms referrable to his cancer and an otherwise limited life expectancy is generally best left alone.

This then is an outline of the advice I would give at present. As progress is made and new information is taken into account, principles of best advice will undoubtedly change. This will be especially true when it becomes possible to predict which cancers will behave aggressively and which will stay as in-situ or latent cancers for many years. It will then be possible to give more definite advice. In the meantime, young men especially would be well advised to take note and learn from the practices of communities with a low incidence of prostate cancer—especially their dietary practices.

Glossary

acute

Sudden; having a sudden, severe and short course.

adenoma

A benign (not malignant or cancerous) tumour in which the cells are derived from glands or from glandular tissues such as the lining of the stomach.

anaemia

A blood condition with reduced numbers of red blood cells and/or in which the amount of haemoglobin is reduced.

anaplasia, anaplastic

More extreme abnormality of cancer cells. Prostate cancer cells are described as anaplastic when they have lost the special and distinctive features that make them recognisable as prostate cells. Anaplastic cells tend to be more aggressively malignant. They more readily invade surrounding tissues and spread more readily to other places to grow as secondary cancers (metastases).

angiostatic and **angiotoxic**

Every cancer and every cancer secondary tumour must have a blood supply to survive. Without a blood supply the cancer cells will die. All cancers therefore develop small new blood vessels (capillaries). A new approach in cancer research is to find drugs or other ways of stopping new capillaries from developing in the cancer and 'feeding' the cancer. The process of stopping new capillaries from developing is described as angiostatic and the process of destroying new capillaries that have developed is described as angiotoxic.

antibody

A type of protein produced by the immune system that recognises invading germs or other substances as foreign. The antibody attaches itself to the invading substance to try to destroy it.

apoptosis

An inbuilt ability of cells to undergo self-destruction after they have served their function. Part of the ageing process of replacement and turnover of ageing cells during normal life. Cancer cells seem to have lost this inbuilt self-limiting life process.

Aredia

A trade name for disodium pamidronate. This is one of the bisphosphonates that give bones some protection from prostate cancer secondaries.

aspiration

Act of sucking up or sucking in or sucking out.

atrophy

Wasting away. Losing special qualities (verb or noun).

benign

Not malignant. Favourable for recovery. Unlikely to be dangerous.

benign prostatic hypertrophy or **hyperplasia**

Enlargement or swelling of the prostate gland due to increased numbers of normal prostate cells and tissues. It is not cancer, simply a big prostate gland, and is common in older men.

biopsy

A small sample of tissue taken to be examined under a microscope.

bisphosphonates

Chemical substances that can help bones resist destruction by metastatic (secondary) prostate cancer. The bisphosphonates become incorporated in the weakened areas of bone, restoring some strength to the bone and resisting further destruction.

brachytherapy

A method of applying radiotherapy by placement of tiny radioactive pellets (seeds) or needles directly into a tumour to destroy it.

cancer

A malignant growth of cells. A continuous, purposeless, unwanted and uncontrolled growth of cells.

capsule

A fibrous or membranous sac that encloses a tissue or organ.

carcinogen

A substance that causes cancer.

carcinoma

A cancer of gland cells or cells lining a hollow organ or duct or skin or other body surface. These are the most common form of cancer.

CAT

See CT.

cell

The structural living unit of which all tissues and organs are composed.

chemotherapy

Treatment with chemical agents or drugs.

chronic

Persisting for a long time. Having a long or protracted course.

closed-circuit perfusion

In cancer treatment, perfusion or closed-circuit perfusion are terms used to describe the use of a pump to provide circulation of fluid through an organ or tissue such as the liver or a limb. The pump system is isolated from the normal body circulation so that the pump only pumps the blood or other fluid through that part of the body, quite separated from the normal blood circulation of the heart and lungs.

congenital

Present from the time of birth.

CT scan (CAT scan or computerised axial tomography)

A method of visualising body tissues by using special computerised radiographic techniques. These give X-ray pictures of sections of body tissues.

cytotoxic

Having a toxic or harmful effect upon cells. Usually used to describe drugs that have an especially toxic effect on cancer cells.

dihydrotestosterone

In men the testes (or testicles) and to a much lesser extent the adrenal glands produce the male hormone testosterone. Some of this testosterone is converted into a very much more active form called dihydrotestosterone. Prostate cancer growth is driven by testosterone but is driven more strongly by dihydrotestosterone.

DNA

Deoxyribonucleic acid; the material from which the body-building genes and chromosomes are made.

DRE (digital rectal examination)
A medical examination in which the doctor inserts a gloved finger through the anus to feel the prostate gland, contents of the rectum, and pelvic organs.

endoscope
An instrument used for visual examination of the interior of hollow organs or the interior of body cavities.

epidemiological
To do with epidemiology.

epidemiology
The branch of medicine dealing with the distribution of disease and causes and spread of diseases.

fascia
Fascia or deep fascia: the fibrous or membranous layer of tissue that covers muscles, nerves and blood vessels, or separates muscles or other tissues into different compartments. Superficial fascia: fat under the skin.

fibroma
A benign (non-cancerous) tumour composed of fibrous tissues and the cells that form fibrous tissue.

finasteride
A medication (brand name Proscar) that blocks the conversion of testosterone to its more active form of dihydrotestosterone. It is given to men with urinary symptoms caused by a non-cancerous enlargement of prostate (prostate hyperplasia). By blocking the conversion of testosterone to its more active form of dihydrotestosterone it reduces some of the stimulus to prostate enlargement and often results in a reduction in size of the prostate gland.

gene
One of the units that make up a chromosome inherited from parents. Each gene is responsible for a different inherited characteristic. Genes are in chromosomes and chromosomes are composed of the DNA material in the nucleus of cells.

gland
A tissue or organ that manufactures and secretes chemical substances necessary for maintenance of normal health and body function.

hormone
A substance that in humans and animals is produced by an endocrine gland (such as the thyroid, pituitary, or adrenal gland) or produced by

another specialised tissue (like the ovary or testis) but is carried by the blood to another tissue or organ where it stimulates special activity or changes structure or function.

hyperplasia

A benign (non-cancerous) enlargement of a tissue or organ. Not a tumour but enlargement due to increased numbers of cells. Hyperplasia of the prostate was previously called benign prostatic hypertrophy.

hypertrophy

Enlargement.

Hytrin

A brand name of terazosin, a muscle-relaxing drug that is often useful in treating benign prostatic hyperplasia. It relaxes the muscle tissue in the prostate gland and at the base of the bladder and this will often allow urine to pass more freely.

immunotherapy

Treatment of disease by giving immune substances or by stimulating the immune system of body defences.

induration

The hardening, thickening or swelling of a tissue or a part of the body such as due to inflammation or infiltration with fluid or with cancer cells.

infiltrating or **invasive**

Describes abnormal entry of a cell or fluid or other material into a tissue where it is not normally present.

infusion

In cancer treatment infusion is the term used to describe the method of adding a constant flow of another fluid to the circulation of blood. Often a type of pump is used.

in situ

In the one place. On the same spot.

irradiation

Exposure to ionising radiation; that is, radiation capable of tearing apart the genetic material in a cell.

isoflavones

A class of plant hormones (phytoestrogens) that are present in many plants but especially plentiful in legume plants like soy. The richest known source is the red clover plant, a legume that contains all the phytoestrogens found to be most active in human physiology.

isotope

Many elements can occur in different forms or isotopes. Some of these forms are radioactive. Minute amounts of radioactive isotopes known to concentrate in certain tissues are used in medicine to allow scans to detect the presence or absence of these tissues in different normal or abnormal parts of the body. For example, certain radioactive isotopes can be used to allow scans to detect the likely presence or absence of cancer cells in bones.

lassitude

Tiredness. A feeling of having no energy.

latent cancer

A tumour with cancer cells that look malignant but in which the cells seem to be relatively inactive. The latent cancer can be there without spreading into other tissues for a long period, often not for several years or possibly never.

legumes

A class of plants that includes all members of the bean and pea families. All plants of this type contain relatively large amounts of the isoflavonoid phytoestrogens.

leucocyte

The 'white' or colourless type of cell that circulates in the blood and is chiefly concerned with defending the body against invasion by foreign organisms or bacteria.

liver

The largest solid organ in the body. It lies in the upper abdomen predominantly on the right side and under cover of the lower right ribs.

lycopene

The natural red colouring matter in certain plants and especially in tomatoes. Diets rich in lycopene may give some protection against prostate cancer.

lymph glands

See lymph nodes. Although commonly called glands, these little structures are not glands and are more correctly called lymph nodes.

lymph nodes

Small bean-shaped masses or nodules of lymphoid tissue normally 1 to 25 mm in diameter. They are scattered along the course of lymph vessels and are often grouped in clusters. They form an important part of the body's defence system. They function as factories for the development of lymphocytes, and filter germs and foreign debris from tissue fluid. Although they are not glands they are commonly referred to as 'lymph glands'.

lymphocyte

One of the types of white cells that circulate in the blood and take part in immune reactions and the body's defence reactions. A type of leucocyte produced by lymph nodes and other lymphoid tissue.

lymphoid tissue

A tissue that is mainly composed of lymphocytes and lymphocyte-forming cells and which therefore is a part of the body's defence system. For example, tonsils and adenoids and lymph nodes are composed predominantly of lymphoid tissue.

lymphoma

A neoplastic disease or cancer of lymphoid tissue.

lymph vessels or **lymphatics**

The small vessels that drain tissue fluid into lymph nodes and inter-connect groups of lymph nodes. Eventually the larger lymph vessels drain this fluid into the blood stream.

malaise

A general feeling of tiredness, lack of energy, and ill-health. Feeling unwell.

malignant

Life-threatening. A condition that in the natural course of events would become progressively worse, resulting in death. A malignant growth or cancer is a growth of unwanted cells that tends to continue growing and to invade and destroy surrounding tissues. It also tends to spread to other parts of the body, causing destruction of other tissues.

metastasis

Metastatic cancer is a secondary growth of malignant cells that has spread from a primary cancer in another part of the body. Commonly called a secondary.

Minipress

Brand name of the muscle-relaxing drug prazosin, which is often helpful in treating urinary problems caused by prostatic hyperplasia. It helps relax muscle tissue in the prostate and at the base of the bladder, allowing urine to pass more freely.

MRI

Magnetic resonance imaging. A technique based on certain genetic laws of physics that allows pictures similar to X-rays or CT scans to be taken of cross-sections of the body, head or limbs.

mutation

A change in a gene or in the genetic material in a cell, which might introduce different structure or function to the growing tissue.

neoplasm

New growth; an abnormal growth of body cells. A neoplasm may be benign (non-cancerous and usually harmless) with limited growth, or malignant (cancer) with continuous, unwanted, unlimited and uncontrolled growth.

oncogene

An abnormal form of a gene that is responsible for cell division and tissue growth or repair. Under some circumstances it may cause continuous cell growth or cancer.

oncology

The study of tumours or the study of patients suffering from tumours.

palliative

Giving relief (palliation); relieving symptoms but not curing the condition.

perfusion

See closed-circuit perfusion.

PET scan

Positron emission tomography. A special technique that gives pictures of different levels of biochemical activity in body tissues.

phytoestrogens

Naturally occurring oestrogen-like hormones present in all plants but in larger quantities in certain leguminous plants such as soya beans. Phytoestrogens are thought to be at least partly responsible for the lower incidence of some diseases (especially of breast and prostate) in people (such as Asians) who have a high intake of legumes in their diets.

platelets

Small disc-shaped particles in the blood that are essential for blood clotting.

polyp

A tumour projecting on a stalk from the mucous membrane lining the cavity of a hollow organ.

prazosin

A muscle-relaxing drug that is often helpful in treating urinary difficulties in men with prostate hyperplasia. Prazosin helps relax muscle tissue in the prostate and in the neck of the bladder, allowing urine to flow more freely.

pre-invasive

Before invasion. In relation to cancer it means a cancer that has not as yet invaded other tissues.

primary or primary cancer

A cancer at its site of origin. A cancer that is present where it began to grow.

Proscar

A brand name for finasteride. This is a drug used to treat men with urinary symptoms due to a large prostate caused by hyperplasia.

prostate

A small gland in males that stimulates spermatozoa to make them fertile in their passage from the testes to the penis. The prostate is about the size of a walnut and is situated at the base of the bladder.

prosthesis

An artificial replacement for a missing part.

prosthetic

To do with a prosthesis.

proto-oncogene

A gene that is responsible for cell division and if changed may become an oncogene responsible for cancer.

PSA

Prostate specific antigens. These enzymes are produced by prostate gland cells and their level in the circulation is measured by a blood test also called the PSA. When the number of prostate gland cells is increased the level of PSA in the blood is usually raised. A high PSA blood level can indicate the presence of prostate cancer, although other non-malignant conditions, especially prostate hyperplasia, can cause a raised PSA level.

radical

Extreme. A radical prostatectomy is removal of the whole prostate gland together with the surrounding capsule (enclosing membrane) and nearby lymph nodes.

radio-opaque material

A substance that does not allow penetration of X-rays. It thus shows as white area on an X-ray film. It is commonly referred to as 'dye'.

radiotherapy

Treatment with X-rays or gamma rays.

red clover

A type of clover plant. A legume that contains the highest known concentration of the isoflavonoid phytoestrogens.

sarcoma

A cancer of connective tissues such as muscle, fat, fascia or bone.

screening test

A relatively simple, safe and easily performed test that can be carried out on large numbers of people to determine whether they are likely to have a cancer or other serious disease.

secondary or **secondary cancer**

A cancer that has spread from its 'primary' or site of origin and is growing in another tissue or organ.

side effect

An effect other than the effect wanted.

sigmoidoscope

A long thin instrument with a light that is passed through the anus to allow visual examination of the inside of the lower bowel.

soy

An extract of the soya bean, rich in phytoestrogens.

soya bean

A commonly eaten plant of the bean family. This type of bean is rich in carbohydrate and protein and contains relatively large quantities of the isoflavonoid phytoestrogens. Soya beans are easily grown and cheaply produced legumes, and form an important part of the staple diets of most Asian communities.

spleen

A solid organ containing many blood vessels, located in the upper left abdomen under the protection of the lower left ribs. Its main function is to filter the bloodstream of old or damaged blood cells.

strontium 89

A radioactive isotope of the metal strontium. Like calcium, strontium accumulates in bone, especially in active areas of bone where cancer cells are growing. The radioactivity of strontium 89 (beta irradiation) destroys nearby cancer cells but does not penetrate into other tissues to cause damage elsewhere.

technetium

A radioactive isotope used in medicine for scanning procedures. Technetium in small doses is taken up and concentrated in certain tissues, especially in bones, in two to three hours. Special scanning equipment allows 'pictures' of the bones in the body to be taken or to be seen on a television screen. In the very small doses used technetium is safe and is soon eliminated from the body.

terazosin

A drug similar to prazosin.

tissue

A layer or group of cells of particular types that together perform a special function.

toxic

Poisonous.

trauma

Injury.

traumatised

Injured.

Trinovin

Brand name of a recently developed Australian product containing concentrated plant isoflavones (phytoestrogens). This tablet is made from the red clover plant.

tumour

A swelling. Commonly used to describe a swelling caused by a growth of cells, a new growth or neoplasm that may (or may not) be a cancer. 'Tumor' is the American spelling.

TUR or **TURP**

Trans-urethral resection of prostate. A surgical procedure in which some prostate tissue is removed by a surgeon using an instrument that is passed through the penis to the region of the prostate gland. At the end of the instrument are a light and a mirror for vision, and a cutting blade or burning loop.

ultrasound

A type of scan that uses echoes of very high frequency and hence inaudible sound waves to form an image. It is useful for studying soft tissues and hollow organs that do not show up on X-rays, and is much cheaper and simpler to perform than tests such as MRI. It is also completely safe to use, even during pregnancy.

urethra

The tube through which urine passes from the bladder through the prostate gland to the penis, and through which sperm pass after they have mixed with prostatic fluid in the prostate gland.

vas deferens

The small tube that transports sperm from each testis to the prostate gland, where it joins the urethra.

vasectomy

Cutting the vas deferens as a form of male contraception.

Viagra

A chemical agent (a drug) developed in America that can aid erection in some, but not all, men who have lost power of erection of the penis.

Further reading

Bishop, J. 1999, *Cancer Facts*, Harwood Academic Publishers, Amsterdam.

Brewer, S. 1999, *Complete Book of Men's Health*, HarperCollins, London.

Frydenberg, M., Giles, G. G., Mameghan, H., Thursfield, V. J., Millar, J., Wheelahan, J. B., Bolton, D. M. & Syne, R. R. 2000, 'Prostate cancer in Victoria 1993: Patterns of reported management', *Medical Journal of Australia*, vol. 172, pp. 271–4.

Gardiner, R. A. 2000, 'Prostate cancer: What should be the sequel to diagnosis', *Medical Journal of Australia*, vol. 172, pp. 256–7.

Liew, L. 1999, *The Natural Estrogen Diet*, Group West Publishers, Berkeley.

Llewellyn-Jones, D. 1999, *Everyman*, Oxford University Press, Oxford.

Morganstern, S. & Abrahams, A. 1998, *The Prostate Source Book*, Lovell House, Los Angeles.

Stephens, F. 1997, *Cancer Explained*, Wakefield Press, Adelaide.

Stephens, F. 1997, 'Phytoestrogens and prostate cancer: Possible preventive role', *Medical Journal of Australia*, vol. 167, pp. 138–40.

Support groups

Several prostate cancer support groups are active in Australia, one or more in each State. They are all integrated with and supported by:

The Prostate Foundation of Australia
PO Box 1332
Lane Cove
New South Wales 1595
Telephone: (02) 9418 7942
Fax: (02) 9420 3635
E-mail: prostate@hotkey.net.au
Internet: http://www.prostate.org.au

Prostate cancer support groups can also be contacted through:

Australian Cancer Society
Level 4
70 William Street
Sydney 2000
Telephone: (02) 9380 9022
Fax: (020 9380 9033
E-mail: acs@cancer.org.au

Web sites

A web search for prostate cancer will find many thousands of sites. Some of these are very technical, some are fringe medicine, but many are directed to providing information and support to men with prostate cancer.

The following are a few sites that may be useful.

http://www.prostate.org.au
Web site for the Prostate Cancer Foundation of Australia, with information about the Foundation, telephone numbers and names to contact support groups throughout Australia, and links to related sites.

http://prostatepointers.org/ww/wwopt.htm
Brief summaries of arguments in favour of the strategy of 'watchful waiting', with references to the printed articles from which these summaries are taken.

http://prostatepointers.org/ww/yestreat.htm
Brief summaries of arguments in favour of aggressive treatment of prostate cancer, with references to the printed articles from which these summaries are taken.

http://www.monash.edu/au/health/pamphlets/prostate
Provides some very basic information and useful links to other sites.

Index

acid phosphatase 51
adenomas 6–7
adrenal glands 12
Africa 7, 19, 20, 27, 45
age:
    and prostate cancer 5, 12–13,
       16, 18–19, 25, 30, 36, 45,
       83–4, 85, 113–15
    and prostate enlargement 2,
       29–30
    and surgery 85, 114
    and treatment 85, 113–15
aggressive cancer/cells 9, 12, 21,
    37, 104, 105, 112–15
AIDS 15, 17
alcohol 21, 90, 102
alkaline phosphatase 51
alternative medicine 25, 103
amputation 80–1
anaemia 30, 35, 51
anaesthetics 32, 39, 48, 54, 56, 59
Anandron 71
anaplasia 9, 84, 113, 114
Androcur 71
angiostatic agents 106
angiotoxic agents 106
animal products 22, 23, 28, 45, 102
anti-androgens 71, 74, 86
antibiotics 33, 40, 48, 56, 80, 87

antibodies 103, 109
anti-cancer agents 106, 109
anti-cancer drugs 71, 74–5, 96, 97,
    98, 105
anus 2, 33
anxiety 40, 100, 101
apoptosis 14, 15, 78, 106, 110
appendicitis 80
Aredia 97
Asia 7, 16, 19, 20, 23, 24, 27, 28,
    45
aspiration cytology 105
asprin 54–5, 91
Australia 5, 20, 91

benign enlargement of the prostate
    6–7, 16, 29–30, 36, 42, 43, 46
benign tumour 6–12, 107
beta irradiation 98
bicalutamide 71
biopsy of the prostate gland 33, 37,
    47–8, 53–4, 78, 83, 84, 105
bisphosphonates 92, 97, 98, 110
bladder 1, 2, 7, 8, 15, 29, 41, 87
    and prostate cancer 46, 50–1
    and radiotherapy 65, 66, 67, 68,
       85
    and surgery 57, 58–9
    and TURP 38, 40–2, 43

131